Hearing the Stream

A SURVIVOR'S JOURNEY INTO THE SISTERHOOD OF BREAST CANCER

Diane Lane Chambers

Foreword by Jodi A. Chambers, M.D., F.A.C.S.

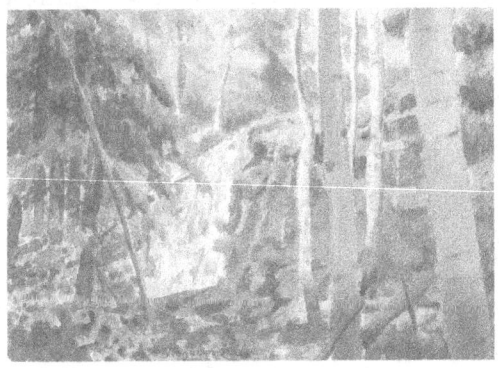

Ellexa Press LLC
Conifer, Colorado

© 2009 Diane Lane Chambers. Printed and bound in the United States of America. All rights reserved. No part of this book may be reproduced or transmitted in any form or by any means, electronic or mechanical, including photocopying, recording, or by an information storage and retrieval system—except by a reviewer who may quote brief passages in a review to be printed in a magazine, newspaper, or on the Web—without permission in writing from the publisher. For information, please contact Ellexa Press LLC, 32262 Steven Way, Conifer, CO 80433; 303-591-1040.

Although the author and publisher have made every effort to ensure the accuracy and completeness of information contained in this book, we assume no responsibility for errors, inaccuracies, omissions, or any inconsistency herein. Any slighting of people, places, or organizations is unintentional.

Cover art: Watercolor painting by Mary Riney

First printing 2009

ISBN 978-0-9760967-1-9
LCCN 2006910198

ATTENTION CORPORATIONS, UNIVERSITIES, COLLEGES, AND PROFESSIONAL ORGANIZATIONS: Quantity discounts are available on bulk purchases of this book for educational, gift purposes, or as premiums for increasing magazine subscriptions or renewals. Special books or book excerpts can also be created to fit specific needs. For information, please contact Ellexa Press LLC, 32262 Steven Way, Conifer, CO 80433; 303-591-1040.

Hearing the Stream

A Survivor's Journey into the Sisterhood of Breast Cancer

Testimonials from Readers

"Harriette and the other women in Ms. Chambers' book provide great inspiration to fight for what we need to eradicate: this terrible disease."
—Karin Decker Noss, late President of the
Virginia Breast Cancer Foundation and
FY08 Dept. of Defense Breast Cancer Research
Program Integration Panel Chair

"I found this book demystifying and a real celebration."
—Lisa Rigsby Petersen, daughter of
Justice Linda T. Palmieri, Denver, Colorado

"Written from the heart and well documented. Mostly, excellent."
—Kelly McAleese, MD, Diagnostic Radiology,
Denver, Colorado

"*Hearing the Stream: A Survivor's Journey into the Sisterhood of Breast Cancer* touches beneath the surface of this disease, sparking smiles and much emotion."
—L. Michelle Bennett, PhD, research scientist, survivor,
and teacher, Potomac, Maryland

"I could not put this book down. *Hearing the Stream* made me appreciate so much more all that you (my sister) went through with cancer and how powerful the bonds become between women who share this awful experience. It is ironic how this terrible disease also has brought so much that is positive into your life."
—Jeanie Silk, Yale University, New Haven, Connecticut

CONTENTS

Acknowledgments vii
Author's Note viii
Foreword ix
Prologue xiii

PART I: AN UNCHOSEN PATH

Chapter 1	Diagnosis	3
Chapter 2	Why?	11
Chapter 3	Decisions	15
Chapter 4	Grounding	27
Chapter 5	Cutting on the Dotted Lines	35
Chapter 6	Healing	41
Chapter 7	Endings and Beginnings	49

PART II: INTO THE SISTERHOOD

Chapter 8	A Journey Begins	59
Chapter 9	Infiltrating Ductal Carcinoma	65
Chapter 10	Prostheses in a Box	73
Chapter 11	Mothers	79
Chapter 12	Prophylactic Mastectomies	93
Chapter 13	Broccoli Sprouts	97
Chapter 14	The Quicker They Grow, the Quicker They Die	101
Chapter 15	No Mention of Reconstruction	105
Chapter 16	Is It Medicine or Is It Art?	111
Chapter 17	Chemo, It's My Lifeline	117
Chapter 18	The Cancer Center	121

Chapter 19	Bone Marrow Transplant Unit	129
Chapter 20	To Lasso a Wild Horse	133
Chapter 21	Terminal	141
Chapter 22	The Miracle Drug	145
Chapter 23	Common Threads	159
Chapter 24	More Worries	165
Chapter 25	Menopause at Twenty-eight	171
Chapter 26	Chemobrain	179
Chapter 27	Arimidex or Taxotere?	183
Chapter 28	Grateful for Birthdays	189
Chapter 29	Peau d'Orange—A Bad Sign	191
Chapter 30	Waiting and Watching the CEA	201
Chapter 31	A Matter of Hope	205
Chapter 32	Burning Questions	209
Chapter 33	Scared	217
Chapter 34	The Power of the Mind	221
Chapter 35	Race for the Cure	229
Chapter 36	We Are Here	235
Chapter 37	Paranoia	237
Chapter 38	Musical Chairs	243
Chapter 39	She's Talking Months	251
Chapter 40	A Second and a Third Opinion	257
Chapter 41	Spa for the Spirit	263
Chapter 42	Friends, Biopsies, Scares, and Loss	269
Chapter 43	Hope and Promise	279
Chapter 44	Sixty Miles toward Conquering Breast Cancer	289
Chapter 45	Blizzard and War	295
Epilogue		305
Notes		307
Bibliography		309
About the Author		311

ACKNOWLEDGMENTS

With heartfelt appreciation, I wish to recognize my editor, Beth Bruno, my family, and the many other contributors and reviewers who lent their time, effort, and support in the writing and production of this book:

Sally Barton, Nancy Beegle, L. Michelle Bennett, Ph.D., Charlie Blosten, Tim Byers, M.D., Heather Chambers, Jim Chambers, Dr. Jodi Chambers, Matthew Chambers, Diane Patricia Chambers, Pat Crawford, Margie Dugan, Jeanna Finch, Foothills Writers critique group, Dr. David Garfield, Ray and Pat Grahn, Cyndi Grober, Harriette Grober, Jeff and Jill Grober, Stanley Grober, Dr. William Haun, Dr. Linda Huang, Dr. Ioana M. Hinshaw, Michael Henry and classmates of Lighthouse Writers, Dr. Lee Jennings, Dr. Robert Jotte, Marie Kriss, Kelly Mack, R.N., Dr. Kelly McAleese, Sara Miller, Mark and Sue Niksic, Karin Noss, Cynthia O'Dell, Sally Palmer, Lisa Rigsby Peterson, Kay Porterfield, John Riedel, David Rigsby, Mary Riney, Chris Schilt, Scott Schilt, Kim Scott, Beverly Shaver, Jean Silk, Vicki Tosher, Anne Weiher, and Meghan Zucker.

I would also like to thank the staff at About Books, Inc. for their fine work, help and guidance in the production of this book.

AUTHOR'S NOTE

With all due respect to family members, physicians, and various other opinions regarding the information included and the events described in this book, I have written from my own perspective and that of others whom I interviewed. The views represented are not meant to be used as guidelines for others who are diagnosed with breast or any other type of cancer. To protect privacy, some names and identifying information of persons in this book have been changed.

FOREWORD

Square Pegs in Round Holes

In the late 1980s, when I was completing my residency in general surgery, breast cancer treatment was an expected part of a general surgery practice. At that time the breast cancer occurrence rate in U.S. women was 1 in 14. Twenty years later, the occurrence rate is now 1 in every 8–9 women. Although that statistic alone might point to a story of failure and despair regarding our progress with this disease, the true picture is actually one of increasing hope and success.

In the nineteen years since I completed my residency, there have been many changes and advances in our understanding of breast cancer and its management, both surgically and medically. I hope the reader noted the use of the term "management." In my opinion, one of the greatest paradigm shifts has been the emerging acceptance that breast surgery and cancer care are not a *single* episode of treatment to be won or lost but rather a combined strategy of management, always with the goal to cure when possible but also to optimize quantity and *quality* of life when a cure does not seem obtainable with today's knowledge and tools. Changes and advances in the last two decades include improvements in technology to aid in earlier detection, image guided biopsies, a greater number of surgical treatment options, immediate reconstruction possibilities, less morbidity associated with lymph node analysis, improvements in radiation therapy delivery, genetic testing, newer drugs, an increasing ability to define each patient's cancer characteristics, and an interest in the merits of complementary therapies. Over the last twenty years we have developed specialties and even sub-specialties in breast cancer care because of the complexity of the disease. The promise of today is an increasing awareness of the importance of integrating specialists into a cohesive team dedicated to optimizing care for the patient.

I am very pleased to be writing this foreword for several reasons. First is to help celebrate the life and lessons of the author, my sister-in-law, Diane Chambers. From the day she was told of her diagnosis to the completion of this book, she has been on a journey. After the initial shock of hearing the words "breast cancer" and her understandable anger ("I will *not* be a victim—one of those 'survivors'. My disease is not cancer!"), she has exhibited a desire to understand all the facets of this disease and to embrace the lessons learned along the way, the lives of others she has encountered, and the preciousness of each and every moment. Second, it is an opportunity for me to acknowledge my patients, both women and men, who have been impacted by the diagnosis of breast cancer and whom I have been given the great honor of accompanying for portions of their respective journeys. Finally, it is an opportunity to share briefly some observations and pearls learned from my nineteen years of being associated with this "sisterhood."

My first pearl is recognizing breast cancer is no more "one" disease than patients are "one" person or carbon copies of each other. Although there are categories and generalities, breast cancer is as unique as the patients who are diagnosed with the disease, and the right treatment for one person may be very different from another. This fact is very important as women and men diagnosed with cancer begin to understand *their* disease and discuss *their* treatment options. Treatment solutions should be tailored to each patient. Any notion of a "one-size-fits-all" treatment for breast cancer would be like attempting to force square pegs into round holes.

Defining the "right" treatment means not only what is surgically and medically sound for the type of disease, but also what is appropriate to each individual patient's tolerance for risk. Breast conservation is a good option for patients whose disease is amenable to this type of treatment *and* can accept the small but real increased risk of recurrent disease within the remaining breast tissue. Prophylactic removal of a non-diseased breast may seem overly aggressive and extreme to one person but is an appropriate and sound choice for another. And whereas reconstruction is a "must" for some, it is not wanted by others. There are two wrong treatment choices in my opinion. The first is underestimating the enemy, treating all breast cancers as if they are the same. The second wrong treatment choice is presuming to know what the patient wants or will tolerate.

When people are told they have (breast) cancer, the shock is numbing and even paralyzing. In my experience patients hear less than 5 percent of what we initially discuss with them because their minds are occupied hearing the words "Oh, my God, I have *cancer.*" Conversations, questions, and answers often need to be repeated, and it can be helpful to have someone with you who can listen and take notes or bring a tape recorder. Most importantly, although patients often feel as if they need to have surgery "tomorrow," they don't. Their disease typically started many months to even years prior to its becoming detectable. There is time to ask questions, get further testing to understand better their specific situations, consider their options, and seek second opinions if there is uncertainty or a need of confirmation.

Increased awareness and dispelling myths are other tools in our arsenal. For example, there is a tendency for people to believe that without a family history of breast cancer there is no risk. This is simply not true. Although having a family history may increase one's relative risk, *not* having one does *not* eliminate the possibility. The most important risk factor in developing breast cancer is having breast tissue, which both women and men have.

My final pearl is one shared with me by my patients—all of them, and it is the paradox that this demon cancer is also a blessing. No one ever wants to hear those words: "You have breast cancer." (No one wants to deliver that message either.) I have witnessed through my patients that their lives and priorities somehow become much clearer after the initial shock wears off. The IDMs ("it doesn't matter") as I call them, no longer orchestrate their lives. The important things—family, friends, love and laughter, things always precious—reclaim center stage. At first blush breast cancer may appear to take something from them, but in actuality patients emerge, whether cured, managed, or fighting for each precious day, as the winners.

Hearing the Stream: A Survivor's Journey into the Sisterhood of Breast Cancer documents such emergence and celebrates the lessons learned in the sisterhood. Thanks to my sister-in-law for asking me to write this foreword and to all of my patients, who have given me a gift by allowing me to share a part of their journey. May the next twenty years see an end to the disease—but not the "sisterhood"!

Jodi A. Chambers, M.D., F.A.C.S.

PROLOGUE

We live near a stream. Each year it rushes with the spring runoff, and every winter it trickles under the ice. My husband Jim and I bought our land in 1975, on Conifer Mountain, because we liked the little stream. The other properties we had considered buying were nice, too, and closer to the highways and the city, but this one had the stream. We loved it right away. We had our own little waterfall and a pond below us, where beavers had built a dam. The property had pines and aspens, and there was no one else around.

Jim and I were newly married and still had our tiny apartment in Denver, where we worked. Every weekend that winter we chopped down trees and stacked wood on our new property. We would use the wood later to heat our home after it was built. During those months, we camped out and slept in a tent.

It would take us a year and a half to build our house, doing it all ourselves on the weekends while living out of a tent. Jim knew how to do everything. He built houses for a living, and he showed me how to help. I remember him drawing a pattern of my feet on paper and sending it to order Sorrel boots from Canada, so my feet would stay warm while we worked through the winter. By the end of the first spring, we had our building site cleared of trees, and Jim called an excavator. We were ready for the foundation and full of dreams for the future.

I have many memories of building our house, but one that stands out concerns something that happened in the early stages. One evening during our first summer, Jim and I drove up to the property together. I'd been working long hours for a couple of weeks and hadn't been there in a while. I was astonished to see our house nearly framed. He had wanted to surprise me, and he did. I was moved to tears because, before that thrilling moment, I hadn't really believed I would have a home in the mountains. I was only twenty-three.

We actually moved into our home before it was totally finished. Then we had our children, Heather and Matthew, and through the ups and downs were happy to be raising them in a beautiful clean environment without pollution or crime. As much as Jim and I, our kids grew up loving this mountain with its abundant wildlife and snow. And although we could not see our stream from the house, we could hear it in the spring, and we celebrated the sound of its rejuvenating rush. It was a constant in our lives.

Life was good. The kids were active in school and sports, and we were very much involved in their lives. But we worked hard, too, he as a contractor and I as a sign language interpreter. It was the path of life I thought we'd be on forever. But as in every life, unexpected events came along. One put me on a new path: I was diagnosed with breast cancer at age forty-six. It was late October, 1999.

The diagnosis came as a total shock. But I was fortunate that the entire ordeal, including treatment, was over in less than six months. At least, I thought it was over on the day the oncologist told me I didn't need chemotherapy. I was ecstatic. I thought I would never think about breast cancer again. I thought I would go back to life as I had known it, not realizing that I had become a different person. My life had changed forever.

Shortly after my recovery, I got a call from Sally Barton at the American Cancer Society, inviting me to their Reach to Recovery training. There, I was surprised to find myself immediately drawn into a sisterhood of breast cancer survivors. I realized right then that even though I was healed, I could never walk away from breast cancer.

Instead, I burrowed in, searching for a deeper understanding of the disease. I read books, went to conferences, and I met many other survivors. Many felt as I did—that sharing our experiences of breast cancer helps others deal with it, too. I seemed driven to write about our experiences. Amazingly, over the next two years, five courageous people allowed me into their personal lives so I could do that.

Through them, my eyes were opened to the complexities of this disease. There was much more to breast cancer than the emotional and medical impact it has on us individually. There were historical, economic, political, and environmental layers that made it a social issue, too. The layers unfolded to me most powerfully as I became particularly close to one woman, Harriette Grober.

In the sisterhood we were all in one boat together, but as my friendship with Harriette developed, I found myself hanging unexpectedly onto her single raft as we sailed over and through the rapids of her harried and intense cancer journey. I was able to witness a life force that keeps people with cancer moving forward, even as options for treatment run out.

It was by these friendships and the power of the sisterhood that, after twenty-eight years of living so close to nature, I came to appreciate our little mountain stream for the significance it held.

Part 1

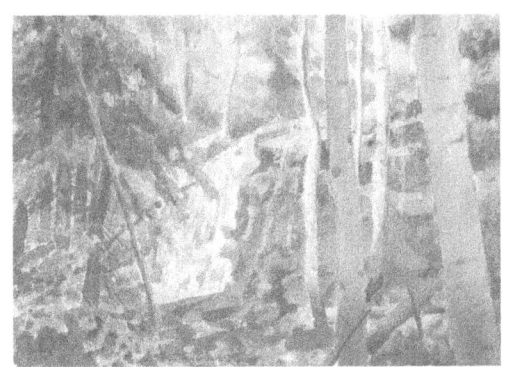

An Unchosen Path

CHAPTER 1

Diagnosis

The day I entered the realm of breast cancer was actually ten months before I was diagnosed. I was in a courtroom where I'd just completed a sign language interpreting assignment at the First Judicial Court of Jefferson County, Colorado. It was December 1998, and I was wondering where Judge Palmieri was. I hadn't seen her there in a while. She was a woman I admired and respected.

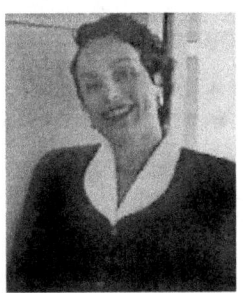

Honorable Linda Theresa Palmieri

"Where's Linda Palmieri?" I asked the magistrate as he signed my "Request for Payment" form at his bench. This was normally *her* courtroom, and I missed her.

"She died," he said. "She had breast cancer."

I was dumbstruck. "That's terrible," I said. "I didn't even know she was sick." He nodded his head sadly and handed me back my form. Linda Palmieri had been gone for a year and a half, and this was now his courtroom.

The news hit me like a ton of bricks. I thought breast cancer was something you read about in newspapers, something that happened to people you didn't know. Besides my grandmother, who had passed away from breast cancer twenty years ago, I couldn't think of anyone else close to me who had died from this disease. But this was Linda Palmieri, and this was bad.

I knew little about breast cancer then. And I knew nothing of the influence this was to have on me. What I did know was a deep sadness and anger, that breast cancer had stolen Linda Palmieri from us. She had been a brilliant and sensitive judge. Whenever I worked in her court, she took measures to respect the deaf person and the interpreting process, which required extra time for our sign language to flow back and forth. She was never impatient or put out with the adaptations she had to make for us. She slowed her normal pace and, though assertive, asked polite questions of the deaf person to make sure the communication had transpired properly.

She had given me a high compliment once when she found out how much I was paid. "You're worth way more than that," she'd said. I didn't know at the time that she had already been recognized by others for her outstanding work. She'd received the Cenikor Award of Excellence in 1992, and in 1996 was chosen as the first recipient of the Anthony F. Greco Award for judicial excellence.

But the magistrate didn't elaborate about Linda Palmieri or her illness when he told me she'd passed away. Subsequently, I turned and slowly walked out of her courtroom. I left the courthouse in a state of shock. In the days that followed, each time I thought of her I got angry at the demon that had stolen her away. I never dreamed I would be diagnosed with the same disease ten months later.

I was standing in the kitchen the day breast cancer changed my life. But it wasn't anger that hit me first. It was denial. Frozen, I held the telephone to my ear.

"We found some microcalcifications on your X-ray. It could mean there's something going on there." It was Dr. McAleese from the Women's Imaging Center. She happened to catch me at home on a Thursday afternoon. Normally, I was in the city, working, but either way, I hadn't been expecting this call.

I didn't know who she was or at first what she was talking about. I didn't know what microcalcifications were. As I struggled to decipher what she was saying, I remembered the routine mammogram I'd had ten days earlier, on October 18th.

"I need to see your previous films," she said, "and if you tell me where you had them done, I'll go pick them up myself." She wanted to compare my last year's films with these recent ones, to see whether the microcalcifications were new. "We need to biopsy this. Can you be here next Wednesday at 4:30?"

I understood now what she wanted. But still, I thought, there was some mistake; she had me mixed up with someone else. I had no suspicious lump, and her assertive demand felt annoying. "Which side are you talking about?" I asked.

"The left side."

I seemed unable to think clearly. My attention immediately went to the lump I'd had for a long time in my *right* armpit, one that came and went with my cycle. "Oh, that. I've had five doctors look at it; it's nothing," I insisted.

"Well, this looks like some calcium, and we need to take a look at it." She reiterated, "Can you be here next Wednesday?"

I wasn't afraid of calcium, and this seemed like an overreaction to me. Nevertheless, I reached for my appointment book. Its faux leather cover peeled away from something sticky on the counter, and I detected the scent of lemon. A thin line of lemonade concentrate had trailed over to the book from an empty can. Ignoring the mess, I flipped the pages to Wednesday, wondering what a biopsy on some calcium would cost. I knew my insurance deductible wouldn't cover it, and I was getting irritated at the idea of having to pay for something unnecessary.

I already had a couple of interpreting assignments scheduled for that day. "I don't know about Wednesday yet," I said.

"Are you not a worrier?"

"Well, not about this," I said. "I'll talk to my husband and get back to you."

"Don't wait too long," was the last thing she said.

I didn't know if I was more annoyed by her phone call or the lemonade-spilling culprit who hadn't cleaned up after himself. I tossed the empty can into the trash and wiped the sticky mess from the counter and my book before I penciled into Wednesday: "4:30 Biopsy."

This was a first. I couldn't remember a medical person ever making an appointment for me that I hadn't requested and then insisting I be there. It had always been *me* asking for something I wanted—a checkup, antibiotics for my sore throat, migraine medicine, or prenatal care. I hadn't anticipated her phone call or the information she was giving me. I didn't have time for this interruption.

It was my son Matthew's senior year, his last season of high school soccer. Besides being engaged with all of his activities, I was taking Spanish lessons, working as an interpreter, and teaching sign language to the Riedel family: John, Mary, and Bert. Teaching them had become a delightful undertaking and my major focus for the last year and a half.

Bert Riedel, an eighty-seven-year-old classical pianist, had become deaf and blind late in life and now lived with his son, John, and daughter-in-law, Mary. Since he'd moved in, the three of them had realized the need to learn sign language. The only way they were able to communicate was through a computer connected to a Braille machine. The machine printed John's and Mary's words out onto a strip of dots that Bert read with his finger. Although the machine served a purpose, relying on it solely had serious drawbacks. When the three of them left on outings, they had no way to communicate except for a crude tapping code they'd developed to answer Bert's questions—one tap for "no" and two taps for "yes."

Their predicament pained me. With sign language, their communication would not have to be this difficult. I immediately wanted to help them. Fortunately, all three were motivated, intelligent, and serious about improving their situation. Soon, I found them to be model students. I was dedicated to helping them learn to communicate hand-to-hand without tapping and without a machine. I spent a lot of time with them, and I'd already seen a major change in Bert. Through touch, he'd regained his personal connection to people. I'd grown to love them, and *this* was what I wanted to be doing.

Instead, I was forced to deal with the issue of Dr. McAleese's phone call, which I hadn't told anyone about except my husband, Jim. I thought up every reason I could think of to get out of having a biopsy I didn't think I needed; however, none of them convinced Jim it was unnecessary. "Just go and do it," he said.

I didn't really believe this could be a cancer, and I didn't think I was afraid, but clearly it was fear driving me. I covered it up with the pretense that if I prepared for the worst, then certainly the worst wouldn't happen. I checked out several books from the library. I read them over the weekend, in between my son's soccer games, and by the day of my appointment I'd learned what microcalcifications were. They were tiny specs of calcium that were sometimes a sign of necrosis—dead tissue. More specifically, they indicated the presence of dead cancer cells. When cancer cells are dividing quickly, the ones in the center die, forming calcium deposits. Armed now with information that I had thought would calm me, I was a wreck. I knew too much.

On Wednesday I reluctantly showed up for my appointment and changed into the pink gown the technician handed me. I held it shut with my arms folded as I followed her into the procedure room. "Can I see my films before we start?" I asked.

"Sure, they're right here," she said, turning on the light tray mounted to the wall. "The calcium is right here." She pointed to some white specs the radiologist had circled in two places. The tiny specs in my breast looked like stars in a dark sky.

"She has awfully good eyes," I said, still doubting the necessity of this procedure.

The technician explained that the procedure for the stereotactic core biopsy would require me to lie perfectly still for forty-five minutes in a prone position on a table with a large square hole cut out of it. My breast would hang down and be locked into a frame while she used a series of X-rays to locate the precise area to be biopsied. The doctor would come in after everything was set. Working under me, she would compress and anesthetize my breast and use the X-ray to guide a long core needle into the area of necrosis.

From the beginning, I felt degraded and claustrophobic. Held tight to the table, my right breast pressed against the soft plastic table, and my cheek pressed against its rim. For a couple of years my neck had bothered me when I'd tried to lie with my head turned that way, and soon my neck stiffened as the female technician worked around me. Her measurements seemed to take forever. While lying down in this unnatural position for such a long time, my anxiety mounted. Since she didn't talk to me, I had to guess when she was finished. At the point when I figured we were just waiting for the doctor, my poor patience wore even more thin. I lifted my head ever so slightly to relieve the cramp in my neck.

The technician screeched, "You moved! Now I have to start all over."

She was clearly upset. I promised not to move again if she could reassure me that the doctor wouldn't be held up somewhere and make me wait too long.

"No, I'll go tell her," she said. After she returned, she began her X-rays and measuring once again. Soon Dr. McAleese came in, which eased my anxiety. She talked me through the whole procedure. Finally, free from the locked frame, I rolled over and pushed myself upright, thinking the technician might apologize for subjecting me to this indignity, but she didn't. So, I apologized to her while she was bandaging my small puncture wound. "I'm sorry I've been so difficult," I said.

She agreed with me. "Yes. It's all right," she said.

I guessed she didn't see locking someone to a table by her breast as demeaning. Admittedly, the procedure wasn't so terrible, but I'd gotten myself so worked up over fear and mistrust that I made it terrible. I stood and stepped away from the table, suddenly feeling lightheaded. When my field of vision blurred and started shrinking into a black hole, I warned the technician before I fell to the floor. "I'm passing out." She quickly helped me back to the table, and Dr. McAleese raced in and raised my feet. It reminded me of when I was eight years old. I had passed out in a doctor's office after I got a shot of penicillin for my strep throat. They brought me back to consciousness with smelling salts.

This time, Dr. McAleese brought me crackers and water and had me lie still until my blood pressure returned to normal. As she talked to me, it was the first time I really got to see what she looked like. Petite with long blond hair clasped behind her back, she walked with a slight limp. She was personable, and I liked her.

As I was leaving, she handed me a business card with the name of a surgeon on it. "You probably won't need this," she said, "because I've done five other biopsies this week, and they've all been benign, but you'll have it just in case." I didn't like hearing this. If her last five had been benign, then the odds were probably not in my favor. Nevertheless, I couldn't imagine that I had cancer. I decided not to worry.

I was home alone when she called with the biopsy results two days later. It was 7:30 in the evening. "It's DCIS," she said, "which stands for ductal carcinoma in situ." I slid onto a chair at the kitchen table. My heart started pounding, and my face grew hot. I couldn't talk. I started writing down everything she said on a piece of lined paper. I'd grabbed it out of habit when the phone rang, but this time I would really need these notes to remember our conversation. My mind was frozen on *carcinoma*.

"The good news is it's in the ducts, and it hasn't spread. The bad news is it's aggressive. I don't think it has been there long."

The pulsing in my head was so loud now I could hardly hear her, but I knew this was mostly bad news. I stabbed my pencil into the wooden table, mouthing a curse word.

"Is anyone there with you?" she asked.

"No. But my husband will be home soon."

"Are you okay? Can you call a neighbor or someone to come and be with you?"

We lived in the mountains on almost four acres. There was no one close by whom I considered calling. "I'm okay. He'll be here soon."

When Jim came home, he found me downstairs sitting on the cedar chest in our bedroom, immobilized by the news. He knew before I told him. He'd read the notes I'd left on the kitchen table.

"We'll fight it," he said. "I'm ready."

The doctor had specified I would need surgery. I was forty-six years old—too young to get breast cancer. What was going to happen to me? How would this affect the kids? How would I tell them—and what about Bert? I needed to see him every week. We had a lot of work to do to get him fluent in sign language. How long was I going to be laid up? Bert was old. He didn't have time to waste, waiting for me while I was dealing with this. Why was this happening now? Was my fate to be the same as Grandma Shaver's and Linda Palmieri's?

CHAPTER 2

Why?

I walked around in a daze for several days with questions swirling in my head and tried to analyze what could have caused this cancer. I needed to know why I got it and where it came from. I knew the risk factors for breast cancer. *Obesity.* I was five foot six, one hundred and twenty-seven pounds, hardly obese. *Heredity.* Neither my mother nor sisters had been diagnosed under the age of fifty, so the signs didn't point to anything inherited. *Alcohol consumption.* I didn't drink. *Hormones.* I'd never taken them. *Never having had children, nor breast-feeding.* I had two children, and I'd breast-fed both of them, fifteen months each. I didn't fit into these risk categories at all.

Had it been my diet? Was it from red meat or fat? I'd always been fairly conscientious about eating plenty of fruits, vegetables, and whole grains and had cut out nearly all sugar from my diet. I'd taken vitamins for years. I remembered how shocked and sad I'd been when I heard Linda McCartney, the wife of Paul McCartney, had died from breast cancer in April of 1998. She'd been a strict vegetarian, who could afford the finest nutrition. If she couldn't prevent or cure her breast cancer, then perhaps diet had nothing to do with this disease.

Perhaps it was from the deodorant I used, or maybe stress had weakened my immune system, allowing an opportunistic cancer cell to proliferate. Looking back on the past year, there'd been plenty of stress in my life. We had sent our daughter, Heather, off to college. I had organized a *sign language only* Silent Weekend for a hundred people, and I was managing our son's competitive soccer team. I always found myself volunteering to organize things, but I never felt I handled the stress of directing them very well.

In recent months there'd been much to contend with regarding Matthew. Although we experienced a hectic senior year with our daughter, his was playing out more so with his objective to play soccer for a division-one college. We'd had to squeeze six out-of-state college visits into his fall schedule and, later, deal with an injury to his leg, which we feared at first might ruin his dream of an athletic scholarship. When it turned out to be no more serious than a bad bruise, we were relieved, but the tension and strain had worn me down. I remembered seeing many soccer moms fuss over their kids' injuries, and I wished I could brag that I was not like those fussy mothers. But I *was* like them.

I was tired and frazzled from the frenetic pace. Besides taking care of my son's needs, I was making travel arrangements for his club team, which was going to San Diego to play in a Thanksgiving Showcase soccer tournament. That's when I first got sick.

"It's a bad cold," I'd told Mary on the phone. "I don't want to give it to Bert." I didn't usually get colds and was distressed over missing a teaching session with Bert. It was the first time I'd canceled, but she understood. Soon after, I missed another day when I was sick with nausea from a migraine. Jim had to call the Riedels for me, to cancel with Bert again.

Fortunately, by the end of October the demands of Matthew's soccer season eased, and I was feeling calm and good again. My head was clear to look ahead to the holiday season. Then, I got the phone call from the radiologist I'd never met.

Five days after Dr. McAleese performed my biopsy I was back in the Women's Imaging Clinic for another mammogram. I'm sure at one point she explained the reason for it, but I couldn't remember why she needed another one. I was in a fog. By then I'd stopped wondering about *why* I had breast cancer. It didn't seem important anymore. We would never know why I got it. What was important was that I had it, and now I had to *do* something about it.

After reviewing my mammogram, Dr. McAleese discussed the surgical options with me. "This is going to save your life," she said. "You can have a total mastectomy, or, if you're interested in conserving your breast, they can do a lumpectomy." To give me an idea of what my breast might look like after a lumpectomy, she gently pulled upward on the area that would be removed. "If you choose a total mastectomy, you might want to consider reconstruction."

Her manner put me at ease, yet it still seemed unreal that it was *me* she was saying these things to. I was concentrating mightily to take everything in when she mentioned the names of a couple of plastic surgeons. One of them was Dr. Linda Huang, whom I was already familiar with through interpreting assignments. I perked up. "Can I have Dr. Huang?"

Reconstruction was no longer something I feared if Dr. Huang would do it. I'd been impressed with her work. Dr. McAleese said she would talk to her, and she would also consult with the general surgeon, who would remove my cancer and possibly my whole breast. It appeared that I had a "team" of doctors on my side now. There were no "why" questions being discussed. There were only what-to-do-next decisions and the question of whether my team would include an oncologist.

CHAPTER 3

Decisions

Since receiving this diagnosis, I'd been handling the disruption to my life pretty much by myself. I told my husband and the doctors that I didn't want to involve anyone else with my problem. I'd had health problems before that I felt had turned into medical fiascos, including one scare with an early stage melanoma and a migraine that ended up costing me $1,000 for the emergency room care. I didn't want to put my family through any more of those. In my mind, this was a problem I could handle alone.

It only took a couple of nights, however, lying awake with visions of cancer ravaging holes through my body, for me to realize this *was* too big for me. I *couldn't* do this alone. I had to ask for help, so I called Jodi, my sister-in-law. She was a respected trauma surgeon and breast cancer specialist in Denver. At seven in the morning, while Matthew slept upstairs and the house was still quiet, I dialed the phone.

"I bet you're calling about plans for Thanksgiving," she guessed.

"No, it's not about that," I said, nervously short of breath. I hushed so Matthew wouldn't hear me if he woke. "I wish it were. I…I've just been diagnosed with breast cancer."

"Oh, Diane." There was a long pause. "Do you have your pathology report?"

I did, and I read it to her. She understood what I did not. "The cells are mixed cribriform and comedo types. The comedo cells are the virulent type, and they fill in the duct aggressively. They're more worrisome," she said.

She explained that the cells were a high nuclear grade and there was necrosis—dead cancer cells. It was an indication that the cells were dividing so rapidly that there was not enough blood supply to feed them. Most likely the dividing cells would break out of the ducts and begin invading the surrounding tissues. I remembered that Dr. McAleese had said the same thing.

"Do the mastectomy," Jodi said. "Your cancer's aggressive and in more than one area. If you choose the lumpectomy, you'll be worrying for the rest of your life about the possibility of cells being left behind. And if the cancer comes back, you'll need another operation."

I told her I would think about the mastectomy, but in actuality, I took her advice immediately. I'd been leaning toward the mastectomy anyway. I knew if I had a lumpectomy I would have to have radiation, and I'd been having flashbacks to my Grandma Shaver. Before she died from her advanced breast cancer in 1980, she'd had radiation to kill the tumors, which had recurred on her skin after her mastectomy. Remembering what Mom had described, I had visions of Grandma's chest as having been burnt black from the radiation.

I didn't know whether techniques for irradiation of cancer had improved since Grandma's time, and even though that was twenty years ago, radiation still sounded horrific to me. So what if I had to wear foam rubber in one side of my bra? I would have the mastectomy. At least it was only the breast I would lose. It wasn't to be the Halstad Radical, the disfiguring surgery that Grandma had endured.

She had her entire breast removed with all of its skin, underlying muscles, and most of the lymph nodes in her armpit, leaving her with a deformed chest wall and lymphedema—uncomfortable swelling in her arm. Back then, doctors believed that removing these surrounding tissues prevented the cancer from spreading throughout the body, but Grandma's cancer spread anyway. Most likely it had already entered her bloodstream before her surgery.

Fortunately for me, this disfiguring procedure was no longer the standard. In 1979 the National Institute of Health deemed a modified radical mastectomy as effective as the Halstad Radical. Thankfully, I would not have to lose any of my chest muscles. I felt sad that this reckoning had come too late for Grandma. But even though I felt more fortunate than Grandma, I suspected if Mom were alive today, she would be heartsick that I was grappling with these decisions. I remembered her taking care of Grandma during her treatment. Mom would come home afterward and break down and cry. Mom vowed, if she ever got breast cancer, she would rent a house on a beach somewhere and live whatever time she had left there. After seeing how Grandma had suffered, Mom didn't want treatment of any kind.

Besides telling Jody, I realized I'd been keeping this diagnosis quiet, hoping for a call from someone saying, "We're so sorry. We've made a terrible mistake. You don't have cancer after all." I would be so relieved; I would say, "Oh, it's no problem. Thank you for the good news." But that call never came. Instead, the doctor's words rang over and over in my mind. *Carcinoma. Aggressive. Multifocal.* The words didn't sound like they belonged to me. I didn't know how I was going to divulge to people, including my siblings, that I had this dreadful thing. In time, though, I saw that denying it was not going to make it go away. I really did have cancer, and I was going to have to tell people.

After speaking with Jodi, I arrived at the Riedel's a half hour early for my teaching session with Bert. I taught him separately now from John and Mary since he learned at a slower pace. John and Mary could learn signs quickly, but without sight and hearing, Bert had to feel every bend and fold of my hand shapes and read the explanations I typed into his Braille machine. Though the process was tedious, Bert thrived on the individual lessons, and we both enjoyed the time thoroughly.

Mary wasn't home, but I found John downstairs in his office, busy at the computer. He worked from home as a healthcare consultant, in a spacious sunlit room where you could look out through floor to ceiling windows into a meadow of wildflowers. You could see Bert's specially designed rope-lined walking path. When Bert was out getting his exercise, John could look up from his work and watch his blind father stepping carefully as he followed the rope, always with Rocky, their Australian shepherd, faithfully by his side.

"Hello," I said, proceeding in. "I have bad news," I blurted out.

John told me later, as I slumped into the chair, that he thought I was going to announce that I was moving. He never expected me to say that I had breast cancer.

He was as shocked as I was by the news. When he eventually caught his breath, he tried to be consoling as I broke into tears. He offered me his shoulder when I admitted my fear about the cancer eating me alive.

I let him know that I hadn't told my kids and that I couldn't tell Matthew—because it was his senior year. Matthew had too many important things going on in his young life. I couldn't add to the pressure. In his wisdom, John got me to change my thinking when he asked me what would happen if I told Matthew.

"I don't know," I said. "I guess he would handle it all right. But how are we going to tell Bert?"

"Mary and I will tell him later," John said, "after we know more."

I thought that was wise. I hated to see Bert worry now over something he could do nothing about, but at the same time I had to tell Matthew. I didn't need to protect my son. Why did we think we were protecting people anyway, by withholding information from them? Wasn't that really more harmful than helpful? It didn't make much sense how our minds worked that way. We wanted to be informed about everything, but then we carefully chose who we told things to—who we thought could handle information and who couldn't.

I would tell my kids when Jim and I could tell them together. We would wait till the following weekend when Heather would be home from college in Durango—another four long days.

In the meantime I was forlorn over how this diagnosis had squelched my idea about making a documentary video of Bert. Since learning his exceptional story, I'd wanted to capture it somehow. As a child, Bert had undetermined hearing and vision problems, but since testing wasn't routine then, he and his family didn't know how different he was from normal children. In spite of his difficulties, he excelled in school and had begun learning the piano as a teen. By midlife his vision had deteriorated greatly. When faces of his loved ones eventually faded into shadows, his problem was finally diagnosed as Usher Syndrome, which today affects thirty to forty thousand people in the United States.[1]

Bert told me that once he learned he was going to lose his hearing as well as his vision, he was in a race against time. "I went to the Zenith dealer and bought the highest quality phonograph money could buy. With my head on a pillow and my ear up close to the speaker, the music poured through me while I imagined myself as the conductor."

He said listening to the music wasn't enough, though. He bought the musical scores of the sonatas and practiced them on his piano over and over, honing each piece until it was embedded into his memory. He would have them forever. Today, in his dark and silent world, Bert only heard the music in his mind when he played.

For the documentary I planned to film vignettes of Bert doing the activities he enjoyed, like playing the piano, lifting weights on his home gym equipment, and swimming laps at the local pool. I wanted to film him taking hikes with his guide friends or Andrea, his attendant, and have animated scenes of them playing Honeymoon Bridge using his Brailled deck of cards. The video would show him interacting with John and Mary and, of course, I wanted to capture our special time together as he learned sign language through touch. The trees, vibrant in fall colors, would be the backdrop for these vignettes. Unfortunately, I needed cancer treatment now, so the film documentary was put on hold.

Jodi called my cell phone at 6:00 that evening when I was on my way to Spanish class. She wanted to know whether I'd made a decision. "Yes. I'm doing the mastectomy." I told her I was comfortable with the decision.

"And you want immediate reconstruction," she declared.

"I do?" Although I'd read about it, I hadn't really thought that part through. Up till now, resolving the dilemma of the mastectomy had been my total focus. I hadn't the mental energy to look beyond that. And I didn't understand yet what reconstruction would mean for me.

"Yes. Otherwise you'll be lopsided and have shoulder problems later on."

My eyes welled up. "I don't want to have cancer," I said.

"Nobody does. But if you have the mastectomy, we'll get to have you around for another twenty years."

When we hung up, I broke down into tears and turned the car around. I couldn't face the all-male group at Spanish class. I drove home instead.

The next morning Jim and I consulted with Dr. Haun, the general surgeon, a sensitive man with white hair. "How are you doing?" he asked.

My lips quivered. "Okay, I guess. I haven't slept for a couple of nights." I was trying not to cry.

"That's understandable," he said. Before I rushed into a mastectomy where he would remove the entire breast, he urged me to have a second biopsy on the other cluster of microcalcifications. "If the second biopsy also shows DCIS, then that rules out the possibility of a lumpectomy. But if it's not, then you could have just the tumor removed with a margin of tissue surrounding it. We might be able to conserve the breast, but that would require radiation. For now, we can't decide anything until you have the second biopsy."

I didn't want to go through another stereotactic procedure. "Can't you just put me out to do the biopsy, and then if it's malignant, go ahead with the mastectomy?" I wanted everything over with, as uncomplicated and as soon as possible. I wanted a one-step procedure. I didn't know this was what feminist activists had fought for years to stop. They believed a woman should have the right to wake up after a biopsy to learn the results. If it revealed a malignancy, she should have time to make her own decisions. The activists didn't like it that women were waking up from a biopsy to find that the *male* surgeon had made the decision and removed her breast.

But Dr. Haun didn't go into that. He just said, "It's not that easy. Before we can proceed, you need to have the biopsy and consult with a radiation oncologist and a plastic surgeon. Then, we'll talk again."

I was already leaning towards the mastectomy, but as I wiped my eyes, I promised him I would make the appointments. I called that afternoon to schedule the second biopsy and the appointment with the radiation oncologist. Most importantly, to me, I also called Dr. Linda Huang.

On Sunday I was cooking dinner when Heather got home. In her ponytail and sweats, she bounced into the kitchen after a long day at the recreation center, where she worked periodically, teaching gymnastics. A former gymnast Heather, unlike most, was tall and lean. People said we looked like sisters although her hair was long and auburn whereas mine was light brown mixed with blond. If you looked carefully enough, you could see the strands of gray that identified me as her mother.

"I'm starving," she exclaimed. "What's for dinner?"

"Lasagna," I said, pulling the steaming pan from the oven. Then she asked me what I was doing the next day.

I hesitated before answering, wondering whether I should tell her. "I'm having a biopsy."

"What's that? Doesn't that mean they're going to cut something?"

I nodded. "They found something on my mammogram."

"Oh." She went silent.

I hurried to get the four of us together at the table in the breakfast nook. The information I had to share was weighing heavily on me. I couldn't carry it any longer. I'd only eaten a couple of bites when it quietly spilled out.

"Tomorrow I'm having a biopsy. The doctor found something on my mammogram, and I'm probably going to have surgery soon."

Everyone was quiet. Then Heather asked, "Is it breast cancer?"

Jim answered her question. "Yes, but they caught it early. Your mother had melanoma before, but she caught that early, too." The kids had been too young to understand what was going on when I'd had that scare in 1987. Hours before I was to undergo surgery for the malignancy on my forearm, including a skin graft from my buttock and a lymph node dissection, Jim's sister, Jodi, discovered an error on the initial pathology report that saved me from the skin graft and the dissection. A misplaced decimal point had led us to believe that my melanoma was much deeper than it really was. With that turn of events, I was much relieved when I woke up from surgery to find that I'd only had a margin of tissue removed from my arm; my buttock had been left intact.

Now Heather started to cry. I looked over at Matthew to see how he was taking the news. He was such a handsome kid. Tall, dark, and lean like his sister, he was in top physical condition from years of playing soccer. He stared straight ahead at the small TV on the shelf behind me; not a muscle flinched. I expected more of a reaction from him, but then he often had his own timeframe for processing things.

We filled the rest of the time at the table with small talk about Heather's friends as if we were afraid to talk about the cancer. An hour later, Matthew came to me while I was ironing.

"Mom, do you really have breast cancer?"

"Yes, I do."

"Well, Tony's mom had breast cancer."

"I know." I had forgotten about this. His friend's mother had been quite sick for almost a year during her chemotherapy, but she had recovered. I had to reassure him that I, too, was going to be all right although I didn't know if I believed it myself. "I should be fine after the surgery."

I found it difficult to tell people about my cancer. Once I did, though, the emotional support I received was most welcome. Since I'd let John know, he and Mary had been great, buoying me up as we continued the sign language lessons at their home. Mary even drove me to the Women's Imaging Clinic to have my second biopsy. The books I'd read said you should bring a friend with you—for moral support and to help you remember what the doctor said. In a more accepting frame of mind, this was a far less traumatic experience.

I understood the importance of the stereotactic core biopsy although I was not yet reflective enough to be thankful for the technology. The first time, my fear had come out in anger and impatience directed at the technician. I regretted that behavior now. Nonetheless, I found something else annoying. With both of us knowing I had cancer, I didn't appreciate her remark after she had bandaged me. She slipped it in on her way out of the room, "Remember, it's all in the attitude."

Perhaps she was hinting that I was starting off my breast cancer journey with a poor attitude. Or perhaps she was just giving me encouragement. Whichever it was, I wanted to say, "Let's cut off your breast and see what kind of attitude you have." But I kept it to myself. I guess I had to be mad at something. Unconsciously, since I needed the doctor on my side, I chose to be mad at the technician. I wondered how much attitude had to do with how cancer behaved anyway.

Later that evening, when Dr. Huang's waiting room was empty, Jim and I sat on a black leather couch in her private office. Dr. Huang had fit us into her full Monday calendar for a consultation. She'd tacked us onto the end of her already long day. After a quick assessment she made her recommendation for my reconstruction. "A LAT flap," she said. "You're fairly well endowed, and you don't have any excess flab on your tummy for me to work with. A TRAM flap wouldn't work for you; I'll use the latissimus muscle from your back."

Many women choose the TRAM flap reconstruction, in which the surgeon removes the transverse rectus abdominus muscle with skin and fat to use in contouring the new breast. Women like this because it gives them a nice "tummy tuck" as well as a natural looking new breast, but I'd read that you're not able to stand up straight for a couple of months afterward. So, I readily accepted Dr. Huang's recommendation.

In my case she would use the thin fan-shaped muscle stretched across my back, the latissimus dorsi. She would create a "tunnel" under my arm to pull the muscle through and position it over my chest. Then she would insert a saline implant underneath. The muscle would give the implant a more natural look and prevent it from poking through the skin. Toward the end of the operation she would sit me up on the operating table. Using gravity to match the symmetry of my breasts, she would fill the implant with saline.

As she sat across from us in her office in a plain black dress that matched her straight black hair, she held a Siltex Saline-Filled Mammary Prosthesis in her hand. "The safety of the silicone gel implant is a controversial subject," she said, "but this one, filled with natural salt water, is totally safe if its silicone shell were to break."

I would learn much later that the cost of this little pouch was an astounding $1,200, but Jim and I weren't thinking about costs then. We were thinking about lessening any potential risk, and we agreed on the saline-filled implant, not silicone. We remembered the media coverage in the early 1990s when so many women with silicone implants had filed lawsuits against the manufacturers. The women claimed the silicone had caused a variety of health problems. The manufacturers settled the lawsuit in 1994 for a total of $4.2 billion. (I didn't learn until a year or more after my surgery that, ironically, after the settlement studies on silicone implants did not show them to be the cause for the sort of ailments about which the women had complained.[2])

I wasn't so worried about the implant anyway. I was nervous about the LAT flap procedure. "Will I still be able to interpret?" I asked. I raised my arms to show her how I use them for signing. She reassured me that I would be fine without the latissimus dorsi.

"Most people don't even notice it," she said.

I prayed she was right. I didn't quite believe she understood how important my arms were to my interpreting work. She handed me an album filled with photos of her patients, showing before and after pictures of their chests. Holding the album on my lap, I flipped through the pages of reconstructed breasts. Some had reconstructed nipples, others didn't. Turning the pages, I tried to remain upbeat and optimistic, reminding myself I had complete confidence in Dr. Huang.

Jim declined to look at the pictures. I was surprised. I thought he would be interested to see what kind of results we might expect, but he couldn't go there. He sat quietly while I finished looking at the photos.

My upbeat attitude crumbled shortly after we left Dr. Huang's office. I'd been trying to be brave about giving up a breast that was part of who I was and a back muscle I'd enjoyed the use of, but riding in Jim's truck on the way home, I broke down into tears. "I can't believe I have to do this."

Then Jim was the upbeat one. He put his hand on my knee, the way he often does when we're driving. "It'll be okay," he said. "You've got Dr. Huang, and that's who you wanted."

To reassure myself, I looked up the function of the latissimus dorsi muscle after we got home. My old anatomy book I'd saved from college said: "to extend and rotate the arm." I still had doubts about my decision, but I had to trust Dr. Huang.

While we waited for the result of the second biopsy, my questions lingered and decisions were up in the air. Should I choose a lumpectomy followed by radiation, or should I have a mastectomy? The mastectomy would eliminate the need for follow-up radiation, which I did not want, but a lumpectomy would preserve my breast and my femininity. Or was I even a candidate for a lumpectomy since there were clusters of possible cancer in two or more places? If I chose a mastectomy, did I want immediate reconstruction or should I wait to make that decision later?

These were life-changing decisions I had to make myself. Dealing with them felt overwhelming, yet surreal at the same time, as I was keeping to my interpreting schedule and performing assignments as usual. My work forced me to put the questions aside so I could focus on my task: taking one person's language and changing it into another's. It required great concentration. I was surprised I could do it, given my state of mind. But I did, and I did it well.

Thankfully, the answer to the questions soon became clear after the second biopsy substantiated more cancer. With DCIS in two places, I was not a candidate for a lumpectomy. I could cancel my appointment with the radiation oncologist.

It was snowing heavily the morning I was to see Dr. Haun again to talk about my decision. I decided to call him instead of driving into the city through a snowstorm. Luckily, he agreed there was no need for me to make the trip. "You're absolutely sure, though, you want the mastectomy?" he asked.

"Yes," I said, "absolutely. And I want immediate reconstruction."

"All right then, my assistant will schedule it."

That lent me a degree of relief since, over the last few weeks, teaching Bert had been the only constant in my life. Everything else felt disrupted. Bert wasn't aware my path had taken this sudden detour. He didn't know about all the doctor appointments and all the books I'd been reading, trying to educate myself. There were so many decisions to make about treatment. I'd never imagined taking this sudden crash course on breast cancer.

Finally, with the treatment decision made, I began to prepare myself for the inevitable mastectomy and reconstruction. I became obsessed with breasts. I was conscious of mine all day long. When I wasn't working, I was either thinking about them or I was reading books about breast cancer. Before my diagnosis, I gave little attention to breasts. Now, I was consumed by them.

CHAPTER 4

Grounding

Thanksgiving was nearing, and still there was no date for my surgery. Three weeks had passed since my diagnosis, and although I'd been reassured that there was no urgency for the mastectomy, I wanted the operation done as soon as possible. The problem with arranging the date was that two doctors had to coordinate their schedules so the mastectomy and reconstruction could be done in one operation.

I was hoping to have it before Thanksgiving, but as it became more apparent that it wouldn't be possible, I grew more anxious. I'd put off telling my siblings and my father about my cancer. I didn't want to tell them until I knew the date. Now I knew they would be expecting to come to my house for the annual holiday feast; they loved to come to the mountains. But I couldn't fathom hosting Thanksgiving in my mental state, and I was agonizing over telling them, "I can't have the dinner at our house because I have cancer."

Imagining their reaction to this news, I dreaded the hysteria that might follow. How could I handle theirs when I was desperately trying to cope with my own? A loving and emotional bunch, my siblings and I tended to carry each other's burdens as if they were our own. I was thankful that Jim respected my need to tell people about my cancer in my own time. He stood patiently by me.

When only five days remained before Thanksgiving, I realized time had run out. I had to inform my siblings because they were trying to make plans. I thought of telling my younger brother, Scott, first because he would be the calmest one. I figured my two sisters would be so frightened and alarmed hearing that I had breast cancer they might become hysterical. I was just getting up the nerve to call each of them when another crisis came up. Dad was having trouble breathing. Scott called from the emergency room at 9:00 in the evening to let me know. He had barely gotten Dad there in time.

Scott, the youngest sibling, had moved back to Denver from Boston six years before to be near our parents. He was the one who had taken on the brunt of responsibility for Mom when she was dying. Now, he was dealing with our ailing father. I pictured this might be the beginning of the end of Dad's life. Dad had always made it clear he was wholly satisfied with the life he'd lived and was not interested in any heroics to save it when his time came. Nevertheless, the doctors were ordering several tests that would take a few days.

With this new urgent situation with Dad, I couldn't drop another bombshell on Scott about me. I only asked, "Do you need me to come to the hospital?"

He thought about the driving distance from my home to the hospital, and given the hour he said, "We're all right for now."

The next morning I called Scott before heading for the hospital. Dad's breathing was improving a bit with medication, but we didn't know how long he would be there. On the phone Scott brought up the subject I had been avoiding. "What are we going to do about Thanksgiving?"

"I don't think we can have it at my house," I said. "They found 'something' on my mammogram, and I might be having surgery." Whether he was alarmed, he didn't show it. He seemed to understand and quickly accepted my explanation.

A few hours later, I met up with him and my sister, Margie, at the hospital. Dad was undergoing an ultrasound, and the three of us stood in the hallway peering through the half-open door to

Dad's room. We hoped to catch a glimpse of the monitor, which might give us a hint of his fate. Chilled and shivering, I was trembling so with the tension of what was to come, not only for Dad but also for me that my sister even noticed.

"You're shaking," Margie said. "Do you want my sweater?"

When I nodded, she took hers off and placed it over my shoulders. She hugged me. I clung to her while she chattered about how much Dad hated all of this. *She doesn't even know about me yet*, I thought, and I clung to her even tighter.

It was later in the day when I told Margie. We were walking to the hospital parking lot, debating what to do about Dad and Thanksgiving, when I mentioned my mammogram results. I said I would be having surgery soon to remove the remaining calcifications. When she finally figured out from my roundabout way that I was having more done than a mere little test, she got more worked up. "Diane, are you having a mastectomy?"

When I admitted I was, she became upset that I hadn't told her sooner. In a heightened voice she cried out, "Why didn't you tell me? I could have been praying for you!" Now she had plenty to pray about.

A couple of days later I was visiting Dad in the hospital when I discovered my two siblings had passed the information on to my older brother, who had passed it on to Dad. "Chris said *you're* going to have some surgery," Dad said. I gulped. I hadn't wanted Dad to know. I didn't mind that Chris had been informed, but I didn't want to burden Dad with *my* problem while he was coping with his own. "He didn't say what for," Dad added.

"Oh…well… it's…breast…" I said. I couldn't say *cancer*.

Dad didn't ask anything more, and we didn't talk about it again. He'd had a sister die with breast cancer at the age of forty-five. I remembered her—platinum-haired, beautiful, and soft-spoken, Aunt Alfreida. I was fourteen when she died.

While I was with Dad, the doctors came and told him the results of the tests. They said he needed surgery to replace a valve in his heart. Without it, they predicted he wouldn't live long. "Thank you for your concern," Dad told them, "but I'm really not interested in surgery." He just wanted to go home.

Soon after that, he was discharged from the hospital. Surprisingly, because he didn't typically take medicines, he agreed to take some at home to reduce the fluid on his lungs. He didn't usually trust drugs or the doctors who prescribed them. He'd seen my mother's suffering and rapid decline with Parkinson's disease, in spite of the drugs and experimental treatments she had taken. He always said about doctors, "They're just practicing."

The finality of his life was certain then, but we didn't know how long he had. The realization that my Dad was going to die was enormous, and in my fragile mental state it was too much to bear. At home I collapsed, sobbing, onto our bedroom floor. I hadn't the emotional strength to deal with my father's passing while handling a major crisis of my own. Jim held me and comforted me in the best way he knew. "This is Bernie's decision," he said, as most of us referred to Dad by his first name. "This is how he wants it."

Jim was right. There was no use trying to talk Dad out of his decision. Only people outside the family tried to do that. The family knew that no one had the power to change Bernie's mind. Knowing that Dad was at peace with it allowed me to let go of that burden.

On Thanksgiving Day, Matthew flew with his soccer team to San Diego for a tournament. The rest of us, except for Dad, went to Jodi's house in Denver. Dad preferred staying home because he thought he would cause a scene. He wouldn't have, but we respected his wishes. We brought him turkey and dessert afterward. I was glad to have the holiday over with. I thought getting over the hurdles of Thanksgiving and telling my family would bring the serenity and freedom from anxiety that I was looking for, but they didn't. I was still searching for grounding.

It was Jim's unwavering strength, John and Mary's support, and dear, sweet Bert that got me through the next anxious weeks while I waited for surgery. What would turn out to be four and a half weeks felt like a couple of months. It wasn't so much that I was scared about the cancer. The biopsies had removed the malignancy, and I knew the mastectomy would take care of any tiny remaining cells, but I was petrified about the operation. I'd dealt with hypoglycemia for years, keeping my blood sugar stable, and I worried it would get out of control in the process. I just wanted the whole thing over with. I wanted the cramp in my chest to go away. It appeared during the long days of waiting. The cramping became worse when I had to talk to people. The pain felt like a heart attack, so I avoided talking to anyone. I was afraid of their questions—afraid because I didn't know the answers. An accompanying knot in my stomach made it hard to eat. Even my favorite foods tasted terrible, and I couldn't force them down. My weight began to drop. I thought I would die from the stress before I ever made it into the operating room.

My struggle about when to tell Bert of the challenge facing me continued. During our lessons I hid my fear, and I hid my sadness about my father. I wanted to protect Bert from the anxiety and pain. As I reflect on it now, I was probably just protecting myself. If I didn't talk about my problems, I could pretend they weren't there. So, I pretended, and John and Mary waited. And we didn't tell Bert.

In the meantime I found our lessons to be a respite from the anxiety. I centered on sign language and teaching. Working with Bert helped to ground me. I felt happy when I was with him. So many times when I arrived from the city, frazzled from the day's race through traffic on interpreting assignments and errands for Jim's construction business, I would find Bert peacefully reading *The New York Times*. He read the news aloud with his permanently-bent index finger moving along the Brailled pages. Other times, he would play "Liebestraum" or "Humoresque" on the piano or practice sign language by himself as he waited for me at his table.

Busy and loud surroundings that incited stress in me didn't touch Bert. His dark and silent world didn't include crowded shopping malls, traffic-jammed highways, or shouting throngs at major events. He had no overhead signs or magazine stands competing for his attention, no television sensationalizing the latest story. Bert did not have to contend with society in the manner in which most of us did. On that level his world was more tranquil. And when I was with him, he brought me into that serene world. The deaf-blind world, without accoutrements, strips us down to the bare essence of our humanity, to important things such as human touch and communication. In some ways it was a gift.

Although Bert grounded me with a serenity we hearing folks are not privy to, I knew he had his own challenges. In his blindness he had barriers to objects, but with his deafness, he had barriers to people and communication. For social beings, as we are, this was huge. Although he was able to keep up with world news through *The New York Times*, he got his news weeks later than everyone else. Locally, he had little means of knowing what was happening in his own town or right outside his door. He couldn't even look out his own window to know what the weather was doing. "Is it snowing outside?" he would ask me. "Without the sun's warmth on my skin, I can't even tell if it's day or night."

Every day I saw how Bert dealt with his challenges, his barriers, and his adversity. I remembered how our sign language lessons had become disrupted when he broke his neck and wrist shortly after I met him. A misplaced foot on a staircase had sent him tumbling to the bottom landing. Mary saved his life that day when she signed "*Stop*" into his hand. New to sign language as she was, it was the only sign she could think to sign to him so he wouldn't move. If he had, he might have severed the nerve in his neck that controlled his breathing. After the fall, he was not only blind and deaf but confined to a heavy metal halo screwed into his skull. Then he was moved from the hospital to a life care center where he underwent rehabilitation.

In these often-impersonal institutions Bert worked to regain his strength. Fortunately, I was in contact with him during his hospital stay, but it was not until he was moved to the life care center that we were able to resume our sign language lessons. It impressed me that, even in the stiff metal halo, he never gave up trying to understand my hand movements, no matter how difficult he found them. He persevered, trying to read each shape of my hand with his fingers, translating signs he could not see into words he could not hear.

In spite of the confines of the nursing home and the halo, Bert was determined to play his piano each day. He played the tunes he had lodged in his memory; the music he could only feel. Never did he miss a note. After his fracture had healed and he had moved back home, I often left their house with the picture of him, his fluffy white hair and plaid flannel shirt in my mind and the sounds of Beethoven or Bach in my head.

With Bert, my stress evaporated. We laughed and we talked. We worked hard and we played hard. Time with him helped me to slow down and appreciate the simple, most precious things. I always left him with a new lightness in my step. But now I had breast cancer and my world had been turned upside down. I didn't want Bert's world to be turned upside down, too, so I didn't tell him about mine.

CHAPTER 5

Cutting on the Dotted Lines

Thanksgiving had come and gone, but my angst continued. Even learning that the surgery date was set for November 30th didn't relieve the cramp in my chest. I was counting the hours. When there were only twenty-four left to go, Dr. Huang wanted me to come to her office to sign the consent forms for surgery. It felt good to be moving forward, and during the hour drive there, I just wanted to keep moving. I wanted all of this over with, but I had to stop for gas. As the tank filled, I realized the tires on my Outback looked awfully low. The air gauge registered only twenty-five pounds each in two of the tires. I thought they were supposed to have thirty-two. I pulled the air hose around to each tire, and as I pulled, the cramp in my chest tightened. I worried it was my heart.

The cramping persisted while I waited in a blue paper gown for Dr. Huang. Her nurse entered the small examination room carrying a prescription pad. "You'll need to take ten days of oral antibiotics when you get home from the hospital," she said. She wrote down the prescription and ripped the paper from the pad. "Can you take Percocet for the post-surgical pain?"

"I'd rather have Vicodin," I said as my hand found the tightening place near my heart. "But right now I'm having pain right here."

She wrinkled her brow and stopped writing. "You better let Dr. Huang know about that."

Dr. Huang shared the same concerned expression when I told her about my chest pain. "It's probably just anxiety," she said with no offer as to what I should do about it. Perhaps she didn't know what to do about my mental state, but she did know what to do with the black permanent marker she held in her hand. She pulled my blue paper gown aside and began drawing dotted lines around my left nipple.

"These are for Dr. Haun, so he knows where to cut tomorrow," she said. She lifted my arm and drew a two-inch dotted line in my left axilla and then started to draw a six-inch elliptical circle on my back. "I know how badly you scar," she said, referring to my old keloids, "so we'll try to make the incisions as few and as small as possible." Where most people's surgical scars heal into thin white lines that fade away, my scars turned red and tended to thicken. They grew wide and raised. Over time some of mine had turned white and smooth but were still wide. I appreciated how she was mindful. That night, I showed Jim her line drawings on my body. We couldn't speak the words of what we were feeling then, but our tender intimacy spoke them.

I slept little that night and was happy to see morning, when we were finally on our way to the hospital. I was looking forward to the anesthesia to take me away for some much-needed sleep. While Jim drove, the acute pain in my chest subsided at last. It seemed my fear had melted away.

Jim stayed with me in the pre-op area where the nurse started my IVs. He had brought his leather portfolio and cell phone so he could get some work done while he was away from his job site. As the owner of the business, it was rare that he took time away from work. The only occasions he missed work were for weddings, funerals, or the kids' athletic competitions. "You can go back to work while I'm asleep," I told him. "It's going to be a long operation."

"No," he said. He would sit in the waiting room with his mother.

My mastectomy was scheduled for 2:30 in the afternoon. Dr. Linda Huang would not start the reconstruction until 4:30, after Dr. Haun had removed my cancerous breast. I hoped she wouldn't be too tired, starting that late in the day.

A minute before 2:30 the anesthesiologist pushed a syringe of Tagamet into my IV. The medicine, intended to decrease stomach acid and fluid, created a wave of nausea, to where I could no longer sit up on the gurney. As I lay back, I said to Jim, "Just remember if anything happens to me in there, I really love you." And then I was out. The propofol had put me to sleep.

"Open your eyes," was the first thing I heard when I woke. "The surgery's all finished."

"Already?" I said in a rough scratchy voice. The six-hour surgery had felt like five minutes. "That was fast." I could hardly get the words out. My voice was hoarse from the breathing tube that had just been removed from my airway. A machine had been keeping me breathing during the operation because of a drug that had paralyzed my muscles. The drug had prevented me from moving or coughing by paralyzing my diaphragm. But I was breathing on my own now.

"We're taking you to your room," the woman said.

I felt incredible hunger pangs. "I'm starving," I groaned.

She laughed. "Nobody ever says *that* when they first wake up."

The only pain I felt was a burning at the small of my back where the doctor had detached the latissimus dorsi muscle to use in the reconstruction. Everything else was numb. And I was coherent enough to look under my gown at my breasts. What I saw was immediately reassuring. There were two, and I was happy. I was happy to see Jim, too.

"Dr. Huang said you did great. She looked exhausted. I'm exhausted, too," he said. "It's 9:30, and I'm going home."

The next forty-eight hours were a blur of people, intense headaches, and vomiting. At one point I looked through the blur and caught a nurse's face looking down at me.

"Haven't you been emptying these drains?" she asked.

"What drains?" I said. I hadn't been aware of them.

"These. Jackson Pratt drains." She had my gown pulled up, revealing two tubes with pouches on the ends. One hung from my rib and the other from my armpit. No one had told me about them although I knew from the books they were there to drain the fluid accumulating in the wounds. "You're supposed to be emptying them yourself."

I was a little shocked at her scolding. I still had a catheter and hadn't even been out of bed yet. Then Dr. Haun came to see me. He simply asked how I was doing, and I fell to tears. I could only whisper, "I'm…so…overwhelmed." I needed someone to hold me and tell me everything was okay, that it was normal to be overwhelmed. Instead, a nurse brought me Valium.

Jim's mother, Palma, a retired nurse, came to the hospital. She came every day for the four days I was there and sat with me. She waited long hours, hoping to see the doctor who would give us my pathology report, but he never came while she was there. Other people came, too: Jim's sister Jodi, my sister Margie, my brother Scott, and a technician, who came in every two hours to check my vital signs. A chaplain came and a dietician. I would ask each person I didn't recognize, "Are you a nurse?" When the person said no, I had no interest in him or her. I had a terrible headache, and I just wanted a nurse, but nurses were in short supply.

A young woman in a business skirt came in, but I couldn't focus on what she said. I was feeling sick. I looked at her and said, "I'm going to throw up." Horror crossed her face. "I'll just leave my business card," she said. Quickly placing it on my bedside table, she ran from the room. I threw up all over my bed. I felt for the nurse's call button. It seemed like fifteen minutes while I lay in my own vomit until a nurse came with an aide trailing behind her. She was shocked to see me lying with my hair in the mess.

"Diane, I didn't know you were sick," she gasped. She helped me up to a chair while an aide changed my bed. "You can clean your hair over there," the aide said, pointing to the sink with no offer of help. Days later, I would look for the business card of the young woman who had visited, but it was gone. I never found out who she was or what she had wanted to do for me.

When my day-nurse was too busy with her twenty-eight other patients, Palma saw to my needs. When I broke out madly itching all over my body, she called the nurse.

"It's from the morphine," the nurse said. "I'll bring some Benadryl."

On the second day after surgery, Palma helped me to a chair when my lunch tray arrived. But I started to pass out in the chair, and she had to help me back to the bed. When I was too sick to eat the hospital food, she found fresh strawberries for me and cottage cheese.

When I finally did get out of the bed, I thought I should walk. I'd had too many drugs and wanted them out of my system. The sooner I got up and began moving around, I believed, the quicker I would recover. Years before, when my children had been born by Cesarean sections, I remembered the nurses had made me get up and walk exactly twenty-four hours after the surgery. I was mad at them because I didn't feel ready to get up. They were right, though. It made me recover faster. Now, the nurses acted like I was crazy for wanting to walk.

"You've just had two major surgeries. It's okay to rest," they said. But I walked anyway, with Palma. We walked once up the hallway and back down.

That night it started snowing, and Jim called from home in Conifer instead of driving to the hospital to visit me. "I hope it's okay if I don't come," he said. "The roads are pretty bad."

"It's okay," I said. "You better stay home."

He wanted to know whether I would be getting out of the hospital in the morning. "I'll come tomorrow to pick you up."

"I'm not ready to come home yet," I said. "I can't take care of myself." I knew he would have to be at work since he was against a deadline on his construction project. His clients were expecting him to have their home completed for them to move into in a few short weeks. At home our bedroom was in the basement, far from the kitchen, and I would have no one there to help me.

Dr. Huang made her rounds the next morning in spite of the continuing snowstorm. I pleaded with her to let me stay one more day although later I had regrets. The sounds coming from the hallways and the PA system were becoming increasingly disturbing and frightening. "*Cor-zero*, room four, *respiratory*, room seven, *stat*. We need a cardiologist in room nine *immediately*." A woman in agonizing pain was the final straw for me. As her chilling screams streamed through the hallways, I asked my nurse, "What's the matter with her?"

"They're changing her bandages, and it hurts when her wounds are exposed to the air."

I was horrified imagining what the poor woman was having to endure. It was upsetting that people were sick and dying all around me. I didn't think I belonged in the hospital anymore, and I wanted out. The next morning, I began dressing to go home. I'd brought some elasticized sweatpants and a flannel shirt that buttoned up the front, just like the books suggested. It will be too difficult to raise your arms and pull a shirt over your head, the books said, and the surgical area will be uncomfortable and swollen. I didn't normally wear these kinds of boxy, shapeless clothes, and they depressed me. I tried to think positively about it, but I didn't know what to do about my bra. There was no way to put mine on over the bandages and drains, and my muscle had swollen over the implant. Since the age of thirteen, I'd never gone without a bra.

Jim arrived just after I'd pulled on the sweatpants and found me lying in a heap on the bed, crying. I'd become too exhausted just trying to get dressed.

"I don't know what to do about this," I said wistfully, dangling my bra.

"Don't worry about it," he said.

I would eventually resolve my dilemma about the bra, but for now it felt degrading to be going home braless. Jim had taken the day off to bring me home, and he would devote the entire weekend to taking care of me. At home there were bouquets of flowers, cards, and letters, including one from Bert, in which he wrote, "One does not truly appreciate the value of a great friend until there is an interruption in that relationship." He said he would never forget that I had helped breathe life back into him by teaching him sign language and through touch had helped him reconnect to humans. I would soon see how he, too, gave life back to me.

After reading the cards, I fell into a sound sleep and didn't wake until evening, famished. Jim sliced some raw carrots for us to eat while we waited for Matthew to bring home a pizza. Thus began my recovery.

CHAPTER 6

Healing

Since all ten of my excised lymph nodes had been clear, there was good reason to celebrate that my cancer was gone. There was no sign the disease had broken out of the milk ducts and nothing to indicate any spread to distant organs. With a tumor of less than one centimeter, this would generally mean my treatment was finished. I could begin my healing. I still had in my mind, however, that Dr. McAleese had said an oncologist might recommend chemotherapy for me. "Each of your tumors is small, but it depends on if he measures them individually, or as a unit, because then yours would measure over 3.5 centimeters," she'd said.

With invasive tumors larger than two centimeters there was more risk for recurrence and spread, and oncologists strongly advised chemotherapy. Since no one can know for sure how any one breast cancer is going to behave, oncologists have to look at each woman's prognostic indicators and then use statistics to make their treatment recommendations. Often, it's a gray area as to whether the uncomfortable side effects of the chemotherapy are worth the benefit, but most doctors like to err on the side of "better safe than sorry," and they typically urge systemic treatment.

I knew my cancer had been a high nuclear grade, in scattered clusters, and the possibility of chemotherapy for me was real. But I had yet to see an oncologist, and it would be several weeks before Dr. Haun would refer me to one. In the meantime I was dealing with the impact of sudden physical debilitation.

The energy and strength I had known all my life had been snuffed out by the surgery. Now my body was using every ounce of energy to heal its wounds. Dressing left me winded. Eating at the table made my heart pound like I'd run a mile. Dishes were too heavy to lift, and doors were too heavy to open. I couldn't let my two ten-year-old dogs, Keisha and Thule, outside. At night, since it hurt to move, I would lie for hours in one position, soaking wet from night sweats. In the morning Jim was gone, and there was no one to change the sheets. I had no energy to make decisions, none to parent my teenage son.

"Can you cut my hair?" was the first thing he'd said when I got home. "Can you sew up these pants? Why are you breathing like that? What's wrong?" he asked. I responded like a zombie in shock. And when I could not drive and could not shop, instead of offering to do errands or pick up groceries, he asked whether he could use my car for his activities. How could he have any understanding of what had happened to me, of what he could not see hidden under my now baggy clothes?

As I worried over my lack of strength and mobility, I felt lost and angry. When I started believing I would never be normal again, I thought of Bert. Suddenly, I felt silly feeling so sorry for myself. Bert would be blind and deaf forever, yet he never acted like he felt sorry for himself. I was not going to be like this forever. I knew right then that I would get through breast cancer.

I spent most of the first week on the couch, as most of my mornings were taken up with bathing and dressing, which wiped me out. When I wasn't napping, I immersed myself in *I'm Not Really Here*, a book by my childhood classmate, Tim Allen. I was thankful to him for the hours in which his humor took me away from my misery.

Palma kindly gave up a week to stay with me at our house in the mountains. She did the cooking and the laundry and took care of our dogs. She also put up with my anger and depression, which were starting to emerge and get dumped onto her since she was the only one there most of the time.

Although I didn't tell her, I hated my new breast, which I thought was too big, and I hated the band of muscle under my arm, which felt uncomfortably thick and conspicuous. Up until now I'd taken for granted the way my arms had always held close to my body, and now one could not. I did confide in my friends, Andrea and Mary, however, about my despair. "I've made a terrible mistake," I told them while lifting my shirt to show them. I thought I'd made the wrong choice of reconstruction. "You go, girl," Andrea said. "You're angry, and that shows you're healing." She recognized a normal part of the grieving process.

My emotional and physical healing weren't totally separate. The large wound on my back, where the muscle had been displaced, curled around to the front across my breastbone. As it began to heal, I felt it constricting. Late one afternoon it seemed to be growing tighter and tighter until I thought I wouldn't be able to breathe. I was near panic. Should I be twisting, stretching, or exercising to avert this? I didn't know what I was supposed to be doing. My mother-in-law, a former nurse, didn't know either. I paged Jodi.

"My chest is getting tighter and tighter," I complained. "Nobody has told me what to do."

"We tried to tell you," she said. "You just haven't been in the receiving mode."

I wondered what else I had been missing for the last month while I had not been in the receiving mode, but later on, after Dr. Huang pulled it out, I realized it had been the plastic tube connected to the drain pouch that was bothering me so much. Beneath the surface of my skin you could feel its ridge running from the wound in the back around to my ribs in front.

The tube was the main source of my discomfort for three weeks—one time excruciatingly so, when Keisha, my lively husky, jumped up on me while I was sitting, eating apple slices from a plate. Going for the apple, she jumped into my lap. Instinctively, I protected my wounds and pushed her away, but her paw had caught in the loop of the drain, and she yanked on it when she went down.

Palma came running when I hollered out in pain. Poor Keisha wondered what she'd done wrong.

Transportation to my post-surgery appointments proved to be quite challenging, too. Each doctor's office was an hour away from my home, and even after nine days I was unable to drive myself there. It required four drivers to get me to and from a couple of appointments one day. My son came home from high school, fifteen minutes from our house, to pick me up during his lunch hour. He drove me back to the school, where we met Jim, who was on a lunch break from work. From there, Jim drove me down to Lakewood, where my brother Scott worked. Then Scott drove me downtown to the doctor's office.

With my poor stamina, just going from car to car was seriously wearing me out by the third move. Scott was concerned before we even got downtown about how I was going to make it through two appointments. When we pulled up in front of the plastic surgeon's office, I pointed to the sign. "The sign says, 'Plastic and Cosmetic Surgery,' but they do boob jobs here," I said. Scott was so surprised I had energy to joke that he burst out laughing.

The appointment with Dr. Huang was enough exertion for me, but I still had to see Dr. Haun. His office was in another building, where Scott and I had a long walk down a hallway. Halfway down the hall, I became dizzy and my heart was pounding. I had to stop. "I can't make it," I puffed. I thought Scott was going to have to track down a wheelchair for me. Instead, I took his arm, and we just walked more slowly.

Although I felt like a train had hit me, the surgeon thought I was doing great for nine days out. We left his office, and I made it as far as a chair in the lobby. "Why don't you wait here," Scott said. "I'll bring the car to the door."

I was grateful for the chair. A woman with grayish white hair sat in one opposite mine. She must have thought something looked wrong with me. "What's the matter, honey?" she asked.

Ordinarily, I did engage in small talk with strangers, but this time I had no desire. I just wanted to sit and rest. In a weak breathy voice I told her, "I've just had surgery."

"Is it cancer?"

I wondered how she knew. "Yes."

"Oh, I know how you feel. I have cancer, too," she said. She began telling me about her cervical cancer. I didn't want to hear about it. I didn't want to talk about cancer. In my vulnerable state I didn't have the physical energy to think about much of anything, let alone the mental energy cancer required.

"There's a cure for cancer, you know," she continued. "It's in Mexico, but the physicians here don't want anyone to know."

I was grateful when my brother pulled up with the car, so I didn't have to debate the politics of cancer with this woman. Scott took me to meet Palma, and she drove me back to Conifer. It started snowing on the way, and the road on our mountain was already snowpacked and icy. I worried about us in her front-wheel-drive vehicle, longing for the security of Jim driving us in our four-wheel-drive Subaru. But we made it home and parked at the top of our driveway. "You won't be able to get your car back up if you drive down," I warned her. The snow on our steep driveway required four-wheel drive to get up. I held her arm, grumpily stepping down in trepidation on the snow and ice. So vulnerable, I hated the thought of falling and tearing something open.

Bert's eighty-eighth birthday party was on December 12. Everyone had hoped I would be able to celebrate it with them, but I was still feeling too fragile to attend. I sent him birthday wishes in a fax translated into Braille.

I felt sorry I'd missed a special event, but I promised I would be at Bert's next birthday party for sure. In the meantime I was trying out various options for my bra dilemma, including sports bras loaned from friends that I couldn't get over my head because I couldn't raise my arms. Even if I could have raised my arms, my pectoral muscles were too weak and sore to pull a sports bra down over the swollen new breast. I finally settled on cutting out the underwire in one of my old bras. I didn't need it on that side anymore since my new breast didn't droop like my other one. The underwire was too uncomfortable now anyway.

I started out thinking this was just a temporary, makeshift measure. Then it sunk in that my real breast was gone—for the rest of my life. A few tears dropped onto a second bra as I cut out its underwire, too.

When John and Mary asked whether they could bring Bert over to visit me, I couldn't say no even though I wanted to. I was so weak that I needed a three-hour nap to prepare for their visit. I was grateful I'd strengthened my legs before the surgery because I needed to rely on them and my right arm to maneuver myself in and out of bed. Pulling my knees up, I pushed with my feet to roll onto my right side, avoiding flexing any back or abdominal muscles. Nylon stitches reinforced the hole where the tube from my one remaining drain exited my ribs. The hole felt like it was ripping open every time I moved. Even slow, concerted movements caused grimaces of pain. Once I was up and standing, walking wasn't so bad.

In the bathroom I unpinned the Jackson Pratt drain pouch from my plaid flannel shirt. It was Jim's shirt. I'd adopted several of his for the time being. The safety pin held the tube and the pouch up under my shirt so they weren't dangling below. When I unbuttoned the shirt, it slid gently from my shoulders and fell to the floor. I had to measure and record the amount of drainage in the pouch before emptying its bloody fluid into the sink. I tried brushing the tangles from my overgrown hair. I was used to cutting it myself, but I couldn't lift my arms to do it now, and I couldn't drive anywhere to go have it done. Discouraged about my life being put on hold, I started crying again.

I was still tearful when I heard footsteps pounding down the stairs to my bedroom. I was expecting Heather. She was coming home from college for Christmas vacation, and she appeared at the doorway.

"Oh, *Mom*," was all she said. She was taken aback, finding me topless, with my surgeon's work exposed, slight and helpless. She hugged me, and I wept, so relieved finally to have her home. "I hate this," I gasped in between sobs. She was crying, too. We held onto each other for a while till we both felt better. I told her that the Riedels were coming over soon. When Matthew came home, the two of them made the house presentable for my friends, who showed up bringing their Christmas cheer.

I was delighted to see that Andrea had come, too. She bounced up the step to my door with Bert right behind her. As he gave me a gentle hug, I managed a smile, thinking that he was the only person I didn't (and didn't have to) remind to "please don't pat my back" when he or she hugged me. It was still too sore.

As I sat signing with Bert and visiting with my friends, I was pleasantly surprised at how good I felt, even festive, with the music they brought. The music was Bert playing his favorite Christmas carols. While I had been in the hospital, Andrea and her husband Rich had helped Bert record it. The CD was a gift for me, a part of Bert I would have forever.

Our little impromptu party ended shortly after he arrived home from work, but even Jim noticed its benefit. After our friends left, he commented, "That was nice of them. They got your spirits back up."

Although I was dealing with the physical effects of surgery and the emotional trauma of what had happened to me, I believed I had been spared the psychological trauma of having a suddenly missing breast. My sense of my femininity remained intact. The only part I had yet to prepare for was what I would see when I removed the bandage from my newly constructed breast. There would be no nipple.

When it happened, about three weeks after the surgery, it didn't shock me at all. I still had all of my normal skin covering the mound, and the round area where I once had a nipple and areola, was replaced with the smooth skin of my latissimus dorsi. The nippleless breast didn't bother Jim either, and though I didn't hate it, I looked forward to having the nipple reconstruction. Each time I saw Dr. Huang I would ask her, "When can we do it?" Her answer was always the same. "We have to wait for things to settle."

CHAPTER 7

Endings and Beginnings

Christmas was four days away, and, except for seeing my doctors, I hadn't even been out of the house. I hadn't done any Christmas shopping either. Earlier, none of that had seemed important under the circumstances, but now the holiday was here. Although I wasn't moving very well, I mustered some enthusiasm and recruited Heather to help me go shopping. Because the smallest tasks sapped most of my energy, she drove us to the city and went into the stores while I waited in the car. The cold was bitter, and I sat wrapped in a blanket, trying to stay cozy in the parking lot of Bed Bath & Beyond.

I had just opened a book when Heather came hurrying back to the car. She needed me to come in to the store. "I don't know if I picked out the right stuff, and they won't let me use your credit card," she said.

I tried to keep up with her walking across the parking lot, but I couldn't. The cold caused a spasm in the transplanted muscle on my chest. It felt like the muscle was going to rip my chest apart, trying to go back to the place whence it came. Breathing competed with walking.

"Mom, you're so slow."

"Yeah…I know."

We started laughing because when she was younger, she used to complain I walked too fast. She said I embarrassed her. Now I was too slow. I barely had the breath to laugh. All I could do was stand in place. It hurt too much to walk and laugh at the same time, but I made it into the store to where she had left her shopping cart and selections. "These are fine," I said. "Let's pay and get out."

Heather wrapped all the gifts when we got home and arranged them around the tree. I had decorated it the day after Thanksgiving, trying to distract myself from the upcoming operation.

I was thankful that I could see my dad on Christmas day. Although we usually celebrated Christmas at our house, this year we drove down to the city so that his weak heart wouldn't have to deal with coming up to our high altitude. Everyone was aware that this was likely to be the last family gathering with our father, and I was happy I could be part of it. I felt bad that I hadn't been available to lend him support. Now we just held each other. We didn't know what to say.

A few days later I managed some errands when Heather drove me to Alfalfa's. I thought I deserved something "good" for myself, so I wanted to buy a special calendula cream to rub on my scars. Calendula was supposedly good for softening scars, and I was concerned about mine becoming keloid.

I asked a store clerk to help us locate the calendula cream. When she tried to offer me a substitute, I mentioned to her that I'd just had surgery for breast cancer and I specifically wanted calendula cream—for my scars. "I have breast cancer, too," she said, "only I'm choosing not to treat it. My mother and my sister both had breast cancer and conventional treatment, and they both died. I refuse to do it."

I couldn't imagine someone walking around *alive* with active breast cancer talking so nonchalantly. "What do you mean you *have* breast cancer?" I asked.

"I have two tumors, but they're shrinking."

"How's that happening?"

"I take this." She reached out and grasped two bottles of IP-6 from the shelf and handed them to me. "Hold on," she said. "I'll get you a book about it." She gave me a small paperback to take home and read. I carried it home along with the calendula cream we found. Sometime later, I decided it couldn't hurt to boost myself with IP-6, too, and I bought a stash of the supplements and started taking them religiously.

As the year ended, I felt I'd made significant strides in my recovery. Although I still couldn't twist and turn well enough to drive, I wanted to resume teaching Bert. So, on New Year's Day, Andrea brought him to my house. Bert didn't often get invited out, so it was a treat for him. He was more jovial than ever that day. My dogs were equally delighted in Bert, as they discovered he kept doggie treats in his pocket. They enjoyed some fun together before I tried to get Bert's attention onto a sign language lesson, but then it seemed Bert wasn't really interested in working on sign language. He said, "Let's dance."

"Dance?" I repeated. I'd never danced with a deaf-blind man before.

"Yes," he said. "Let's celebrate the New Year."

So, while Andrea and my dogs watched, I led him to a space in front of our Christmas tree. We stood swaying back and forth while the colored lights blinked and Bert sang "Auld Lang Syne." I thought dancing with Bert was the perfect way to begin a new year—a year without breast cancer.

As my life began anew, my father's ended. He passed away six days after the New Year, less than one day after my brother Chris flew in from Arizona and my sister Jeanie from Connecticut. They came out in a hurry when we knew his death was imminent. We gathered together at the Hospice during Dad's last hours when he was heavily medicated on morphine. I broke down and cried in my brother's arms. "I hate seeing him this way," I said. He was battered and bruised from a bad reaction he'd had to Ativan. It'd made him so crazy and violent that five security guards had to fight him down and restrain him. The doctors had to increase the dose to where he'd become unconscious. I knew Dad never wanted to be drugged in this way, but it was the only means of easing him over to the "other side" while he was struggling to breathe.

More than one hundred people came to the memorial service and catered reception we held two days later. My siblings had organized it that quickly. It was overwhelming for me to see that so many people cared about Dad, who was the stay-at-home type and rarely strayed from his routine. Many of the people I hadn't seen in years, and I was so excited to see each of them that I couldn't focus on the sadness of losing Dad. Instead, it seemed like a celebration, and I guess it was. We were celebrating Dad, and I was celebrating my recovery as well. I tried to talk to each person at the reception, but as the afternoon stretched into the evening hours, I grew lifeless from exhaustion and asked Jim to take us home. I fell asleep in the car.

The next day Heather drove me back to the city, and again each day for the next five so I could be with my siblings while we cleared out Dad's house and settled his affairs. Like five "chiefs" we each took on tasks. Watching them run circles around me, I became aware of how much further I still had to go in my recovery. They cleaned out drawers, closets, and cabinets while I could only sit. I went through Dad's papers and old photos.

One task, however, was my sole responsibility. Scott drove me to the bank where Dad kept his safety deposit box. On the way there I took the key from my purse, where I'd kept it safe for several years. "I can't believe this day has actually come," I said. "I remember the day he gave me this key and brought me to see what he had in the box. He said, 'When I go, all the papers you'll need are right here.'" Dad had all of his affairs in exact order for us—ready for this day. I started to cry when I handed the key to the bank employee. "We're here to empty my dad's box," I told her. Losing Dad was sad, but being close to my siblings that week was one of the most wonderfully special times in my life.

Up until then I had been continuing to obsess about breasts and read every book I could find on breast cancer. I was still worrying over whether I would need to take chemotherapy, which I really didn't want. I was scared of it, and Jim saw me getting freaked out repeatedly by the books I was reading. Some were medical texts and others were women's personal stories. They each carried a grim message, and I would wonder whether I was headed down a dark road. But Jim was optimistic. "You're going to be fine," he said. "Stop reading those books." I'd put one down only to pick it back up fifteen minutes later and start reading again.

I couldn't seem to get on with my life until I knew for certain that I was finished with treatment and could put the cancer behind me. My obsessing finally did come to a halt. The turning point was when the words I'd been waiting to hear for nearly three months came from the oncologist.

I sat across from him in his small paper-cluttered office. "You don't need chemotherapy," he said, reading my files. With no positive nodes or sign of invasion, he had no reason to believe that any stray microscopic cells were floating around in my body. The protocol called for no further treatment. "And there's no indication tamoxifen will benefit you, either." He told me that he'd made his assessment on the computer using my personal and family history to make his determination. "You're of low risk."

I was glad to hear this. I hadn't wanted to take tamoxifen. The drug is often recommended after a breast cancer diagnosis because it can reduce the risk of a new cancer in the opposite breast. It's a good drug, but like all drugs it has potential risks and side effects, too. The one I would later hear most women complain about is hot flashes, but other possibilities included vaginal dryness, sexual dysfunction, phlebitis, pulmonary embolism, retinopathy, and even endometrial cancer. I guessed that the oncologist believed that, because I was of low enough risk, these side effects were simply not worth the uncertain benefit.

The hour consultation cinched it. I'd dwelled on cancer long enough. I'd had a successful mastectomy, recovered from reconstructive surgery, and heard what I wanted to hear. I'd survived. "Thank you," I said, with a sigh of relief. With lighter steps, I was on my way.

I went back to work interpreting, and by early spring felt like a normal person again. The swelling had gone down, and I was eager to get my nipple. Through my T-shirts, I could see *one* on my chest, but I wanted *two*. I knew that many women who have reconstruction after mastectomies forgo the nipple reconstruction because they're either comfortable with what they have or they don't want any more surgery. But I wanted it, and I was excited about having cosmetic surgery, not anxious like I was for the mastectomy.

In March Dr. Huang finally agreed "things looked settled" and we could go ahead with the last part of the reconstruction. She fashioned the nipple from the skin tissue that was covering the hole left by my original nipple. In the first operation she had carefully tucked the skin flap under my "spared" breast skin, so she could use it later. Now she pulled the skin up to form the knot that resembled a real nipple. Later that summer, after it had healed, I had the new nipple and areola tattooed with a dark color to match my natural one. I was a happy girl.

I knew I'd been lucky. Because my cancer had been diagnosed at an early stage, I had not suffered the same fate as my grandmother and Linda Palmieri. I was aware, however, that my experience was not the same as many other's. Still, I wanted the entire ordeal behind me. I stopped thinking about breasts. I took my new energy and put it into writing. Jim bought me a new computer, and I signed up for a computer class. I signed up for writing classes, and I joined two writers' groups. I began meeting a world of new friends. I didn't think about cancer any more or about my breasts, until the fall when I went swimming.

Swimming had been a part of my life since I was a seven-year-old peewee on the Congress Park swim team. I competed every summer and all through high school. Later, I taught swimming lessons and, before I was married, had even been a lifeguard. Since my operation, however, I hadn't even tried a bathing suit on. But, while Jim and I were in New Hampshire visiting our son in college, I felt motivated to take a dip in the hotel pool. Before breakfast I slipped out of my nightgown into my suit and stood hesitantly before him.

"The scars don't even show," Jim said. "No one can tell."

We were both pleased to see I looked no different than before. Now, I needed to see whether I could still swim. Since Jim didn't enjoy swimming the way I did, I went by myself.

It felt great to be in a pool again. I was totally alone, and the water felt invigorating. I submerged my head and started the crawl down the length of the pool. By the first pull, I could feel the difference on my left side. My arm was considerably weaker without the latissimus to pull back on the water, yet the muscle was still working. It was just that, being on my chest now, it was pulling my breast "sideways." Disappointed and let down, I stood up in the shallow end of the pool. Suddenly tears were running down my face. In an instant the tears for my loss changed to tears of joy—because *I was swimming*. Yes, it felt different, but I could still do it. I swam ten laps, slowly, remembering what I'd heard, *that too much too fast could cause lymphedema*. Still, I felt on top of the world.

Part II

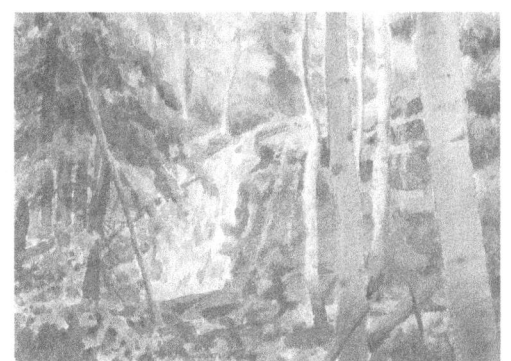

Into the Sisterhood

CHAPTER 8

A Journey Begins

Some people with cancer join support groups to help them cope. But I didn't have cancer anymore, and I wasn't looking for support. I'd read enough books for that, and I wanted nothing more to do with cancer. It had been one year since my diagnosis, and I was back into my old life, life before breast cancer. Soon, however, I found life was different and that after cancer there is only *life after cancer*. For me it was not to be a negative thing, but very much the opposite. It started with a call from Sally Barton.

Sally was a friend of my brother, Scott. She was also a breast cancer survivor and a volunteer for the American Cancer Society. When she heard about me, she thought I'd be good as a volunteer in their outreach program. She invited me to the Reach to Recovery training.

Before this, I hadn't planned on doing anything affiliated with cancer. I only thought about it for a minute before I said, "Sure, I'll come to the training." I would begin to see what *life after cancer* was all about.

Everyone at the training was a breast cancer survivor. There seemed to be so many of us—like when I was pregnant and started noticing all the other pregnant women. Pregnancy seemed like an epidemic. I don't notice pregnant women in the way I used to, but here among survivors, I noticed that all of us had experienced the physical and emotional effects of breast cancer. Now we were learning how to reach out to newly diagnosed women.

I found that Reach to Recovery volunteers understand the fears associated with cancer and the feelings of being overwhelmed, uncertain, and alone. Although the physical effects of breast cancer differ for each of us, the emotional impacts are much the same.

Before I met these women, speaking out about my experience felt lonely. When I told people I'd had breast cancer, they often looked horrified. I sensed their pity for me for what they thought I'd been through. I didn't want them feeling sorry for me. I was not sick and suffering. I felt no connection to them when they began to tell me about someone else they knew who had cancer. They just didn't know what else to say. In my mind, they seemed to understand little about breast cancer and the fact that we don't all have the same experience with it. Many didn't understand that I hadn't lost my hair and why I hadn't needed chemotherapy. I was like those people, too, before I had cancer and before I met other survivors.

With the Reach to Recovery volunteers, I felt a connection. There was no pity among us. I heard their stories about treatments different from mine. Many of us didn't fully understand the differing biology of our cancers, and we wondered about our dissimilar medical treatments. I wanted to know about their chemotherapy and their prostheses, and they wanted to know about my reconstruction and my LAT flap.

But what we all understood very well were the emotions that an estimated 258,000 men and women, newly diagnosed with breast cancer each year, experience. Hearing these women speak out, I was fascinated, and I felt validated. I found the feelings I'd experienced during my nightmare had been normal. But I also realized my experience hadn't been typical of that of many others. My story was only a snapshot of breast cancer, and the whole picture was just beginning to unfold to me.

During the training we learned that our role as Reach to Recovery volunteers was to lend support by allowing the women we would visit to express their fears and concerns, to listen, and to offer them written information about breast cancer. Over time, in meeting with many survivors, I saw how the process of telling our stories puts the experience outside of us and makes it easier to cope with cancer. When we listen, we learn and gain understanding about things that were mysteries before. With understanding, our fear diminishes and turns to hope. Some people join support groups to process what they have been through, and others choose to write. I joined the Association of Breast Cancer Survivors (ABCS), *and* I chose to write.

I went to my first meeting of ABCS in January 2001, shortly after finishing the Reach to Recovery Training. I found another thriving group of women there who had survived breast cancer, too. Joyce Coville, the vice president of the association, welcomed me at once into the group. Right away, I felt comfortable there, like I belonged.

I felt especially connected when I discovered our speaker was a writer and the topic she had come to share with us was something I was familiar with. She came to tell us about her research with the elderly and the secrets she found in how to keep the mind sharp. "I hope you might glean something from my research to use in your recovery from breast cancer," she said.

I listened to her describe a string of characteristics she observed among elderly people, who are still mentally sharp. I pictured Bert.

"The elderly person knows his own body very well and understands how it works best for him," she said. "He maintains an emotional balance by not ruminating in misery, anger, or fear, and he's figured out how to keep on learning. He's found things to do. He has an ability to make decisions, quickly and authoritatively. He doesn't resist change, but embraces it, uses it, and learns from it. And he's passionate about some activity he engages in daily."

She may as well have been describing Bert, who was passionate about learning sign language and was still playing the piano even though he could no longer hear it. As well, he kept up his exercise and visited with friends. Bert was living proof that what she was saying was true. If we keep active and pursue a passion, we thrive. Bert was my role model, and I wanted to be that way when I got old.

It felt good, being able to relate to what she was saying. Afterward, she talked about how writing can be therapeutic, and she gave us a little task. "Just as everyone can remember what they were doing when they heard that President Kennedy had been shot, I'm sure each of you remembers vividly exactly when you got your cancer diagnosis," she said. Then she gave us ten minutes to write freely, whatever came to our minds about that day. When the time was up, we privately shared what we had written with the woman next to us. Joyce and I exchanged papers, and afterward she said, "Wow, I've just met you, but already I feel like I've known you a long time."

Some of the other women even read theirs aloud to the whole group. As I listened, I looked around the room. Spilled tears were not limited to me alone. Most of us were totally surprised by the beautiful prose that had flowed from our pens in those few minutes—thoughts we never knew we had.

I enjoyed my first ABCS meeting. It seemed these women were having fun, and I decided right there, breast cancer's really not so bad. I looked forward to the next time I could be with them, when Joyce said we were going to learn how Feng Shui could help us further our recovery. I didn't know at the time what Feng Shui was, nor did I care. I wasn't particularly concerned about my recovery either. I thought I'd already recovered from breast cancer, but I knew I wanted to be with this group. I saw them as *fun*. I had no idea what this newfound sisterhood was going to mean to me.

Three months later we gathered again at the American Cancer Society. During the introductions I saw there were ten-year, eighteen-year, and twenty-five-year survivors. I was the only fifteen-month survivor. Most of the women were older than my forty-seven years. One was even younger, at thirty-six. And then there was Pat Grahn.

"I'm three months post-surgery," she said, "and I'm on my third round of chemotherapy. I'm seventy-two years old, and a man from my church said to me, 'Why are you fighting this? You've lived a good life.' My doctor has never said that to me. He just explained to me what I needed to do, and I went right along with it. I'm not ready to quit living," she added. Everyone applauded. Pat smiled, and her eyes sparkled under the fisherman's hat she wore to cover her bald head. She seemed so happy to be with us, and I felt immediately drawn to her.

After Pat spoke, Joyce introduced the Feng Shui expert. "Simple changes, like moving a bed, changing the direction you face while sitting at your desk, or adding mirrors can bring you improved health and relationships and increase your happiness and prosperity," she said. I'd never heard of this ancient Chinese art of placement, but if there were simple things I could do to bring balance and harmony to my life, I wanted to know about them. She explained that this method of placing objects and furnishings in our home in a certain way enables the Ch'i, the invisible energy, to circulate freely. "Getting rid of clutter and things that hold bad memories are ways to promote healing," she said. "Or spicing up the entryway with the warm feeling of red can hasten your recovery."

I didn't think painting my entryway red would work for me, but I came away with other ideas about what I could do. I hadn't thought before about how the rooms in my house could be making me feel out of balance, but it made sense. Clutter did make me irritable, and the big junk room downstairs was the worst. It would definitely have to go. But Jim would have to help me with that. For now, to start the invisible energy flow, I could take down the wall hangings in my bedroom. I'd never liked them. And I would quit wearing earrings. I was allergic to their metal, and I'd been fighting the irritation for years. For what?

I would eventually look for other ways to simplify my life, too, but more importantly I came away feeling good about being with people I had something in common with. I'd met survivors who would become very important to me, including Pat Grahn, Joyce Coville, and someone else Joyce introduced to me, Harriette Grober.

The same day I met Pat and Harriette, I told them I was interested in writing and that I'd like to write some women's stories about their breast cancer. That especially interested Harriette because she said she'd always wanted to write her story, but she knew she never would. Both of them expressed interest in my idea about sharing our experiences. So over the coming months, I began to meet with them, as a listener and a conduit for their stories. Later, I would meet with a couple of other young survivors who wanted to share their experiences, too: Kim Scott and my neighbor Sue Niksic.

Over the next two years, as I spent time with each of them, I learned their stories bit by bit. Through them, I began to understand myself better, when I saw how similar we are in how we go through the stages of denial, anger, bargaining, depression, and acceptance—even though our cancers are different and there's not a "one size fits all" in cancer treatment. I saw how these women dealt with their cancer and began to understand what psychological approaches we use to get through the tough parts of surgery, chemotherapy, radiation, and, for Harriette and Sue, recurrences.

As I tried to understand and empathize with their experiences, I found inspiration in how they courageously met the challenges of their cancer. Like a youngster who looks up to teenagers, I considered them to be mentors to me because I knew that someday I could get cancer again. I could be wearing their shoes. Or my sisters, daughter, or friends could.

With time, I learned that breast cancer was not just a disease that affected women. It affected men, too, on the same medical and emotional levels. I would find that breast cancer had social, political, economic, and environmental impacts. We were all affected.

CHAPTER 9

Infiltrating Ductal Carcinoma

In time, I would come to find that Harriette was already well known in the cancer community, but for now I was just beginning to know her. The New York accent was what I noticed initially about her. At least three inches shorter than I, she was physically fit and came across as very self-assured. The first thing she said to me was that she'd been on chemotherapy for nine years. I'd never heard of someone taking chemotherapy for such a long time, and I thought she must be lucky to be alive. She told me this so nonchalantly I felt she held some secret wisdom about life, about how to be happy and thankful for each day. I had no idea then how she would ultimately come to influence me.

We started getting together more, and eventually, over many lunches, I gathered the pieces of her story. She told me she was forty-two years old when she was diagnosed. Like me, she had thought she was going to die. She felt scared and alone at first, but without the compounded surgery I'd had with immediate reconstruction, she was able to heal quickly from her mastectomy. And she made connections early on with other cancer survivors through the American Cancer Society, which, she believed, made a big difference in her recovery.

Unlike mine, however, her diagnosis was a different sort, and it came delayed. Hers was an "infiltrating" ductal carcinoma, which meant huge challenges lay ahead for her.

"It was July of 1983 when I found the lump in my left breast," Harriette said. "At the time, I was working as the executive secretary to the medical director at Craig Hospital in Denver, a job I loved. I was married and had a fourteen-year-old son and an eighteen-year-old disabled daughter. My husband, Stanley, actually discovered the lump first."

During an intimate moment with his wife, he had felt the pea-sized knob near her breastbone. It hadn't been visible on the surface of her breast, so she hadn't noticed it before. "When Stanley found it, he said, 'What's this?' Then, I felt it, too, and instantly the fearful notion flashed through my mind: *What if it's cancer?*

"I already had an appointment scheduled for my yearly gynecological checkup in two more weeks, so I figured I could wait for that appointment to get the lump checked. But all during those two weeks, the same *what if* question kept playing over in my mind.

"On the day of my appointment with the gynecologist, I told him I had found a lump. The doctor found it easily with his fingers, though he didn't seem too concerned about it. He ordered a mammogram anyway, but nothing abnormal showed up on the pictures. Then a few days later, he reported that it was nothing. He said, 'Don't worry.' He was a highly respected doctor, and I trusted him, so I didn't worry."

Harriette occupied herself with her family and her job at the hospital and forgot about the pea-sized lump. She concentrated on her daily workouts at the athletic center. Six months later, though, Harriette found her thoughts drifting back to the lump. She touched her fingers to her chest and pressed into her breast until they touched her chest wall. Then she moved her fingers down a few centimeters and pressed in again, feeling for the pea-sized bump she so vividly remembered. "I found it in the place where I discovered it half a year ago. It felt twice as big as the first time I found it," she said, "though it still wasn't visible from the surface."

Immediately, Harriette made an appointment with her gynecologist to have the lump examined again, but this time her doctor was out of the country. Instead she saw a woman doctor who was covering for him.

"She palpated the bump and read over my records. She even looked at the drawing of it in my chart. The doctor had made notes of its size and location, but since there was no history of cancer in my family and she saw I was athletic and physically fit, she wasn't concerned about the lump either. Again I heard, 'Don't worry. You're fine.' I felt fine too, so I had no reason not to believe her. I didn't worry."

In September of 1984, a year after the discovery of the knob in her breast, Harriette began to realize she was losing weight. "I'd lost about eight pounds, and my clothes were loose. I was actually quite happy about that and was feeling good, except I had a respiratory virus. I still had the virus when I saw my gynecologist again for my routine checkup."

He compared the previous drawings of Harriette's lump to its present size and this time *was* concerned because the lump had grown larger. "He said, 'We need to biopsy this immediately,' and he recommended a surgeon for me to see right away."

The surgeon was concerned, too, because the lump was so hard. "He promptly had his medical assistant schedule me for a biopsy the following week."

The days before the biopsy were terrifying. "Breast cancer was not something people talked about in 1984, and I had no one to turn to for information or support. I was sure my biopsy would show it was cancer and that I was going to die."

In spite of her lingering respiratory virus, Harriette rode with her friend Judy Lezar to the hospital, upset and afraid the procedure might have to be postponed because of her cold. "The doctor was concerned about my cold, too, since it involved some risk with the anesthesia, but we decided to go ahead with it anyway.

"I waited alone for about fifteen minutes in the holding area before they took me into the procedure room, and I started shivering," Harriette said. "The wait seemed like forever, and I was shaking with fear. No one had explained the procedure to me, but I wasn't scared about that; I was scared to death about the cancer. When I got onto the table in the procedure room, the whole thing shook under me, until the anesthesia put me to sleep.

"I did fine, in spite of my cold, and, when I woke up, the doctor said it was black and didn't look good and that he had removed all of it. He said it in such a nonchalant way it was as if he were saying something like, 'Take a left turn here.' He seemed cold and calloused, and I didn't like him. Then he mentioned to me that he'd seen another area in my breast, on the side, that concerned him. I rode home with Judy afterward, bandaged up and feeling sore, to wait for the results."

The following day was Saturday, Yom Kippur, the day when Jews pray together and ask for forgiveness for the last year's sins. "Normally on Yom Kippur we spend the day fasting and attend services at the temple from nine to seven, but we didn't go to the services that day. Stanley and I stayed covered up in bed with Cyndi our daughter lying next to us, waiting for the surgeon to call with the biopsy results. We were going to break the fast later with Judy, but meanwhile we were lying under the blankets, petrified of what the surgeon might say."

Their hearts jumped when the phone rang, but it wasn't the doctor. It was Judy, calling from the temple to see whether Harriette had gotten the results. "I told her we were expecting the call from the doctor."

A half hour later another call sent their blood rushing again. It was Judy, once more, but there was still no news. "The surgeon called at 11:30. He said, 'The biopsy shows cancer—an infiltrating ductal carcinoma, and you need a mastectomy as soon as possible.' The other area in my breast he had been concerned about, fortunately, wasn't cancer, but just the word *infiltrating* was horribly frightening. I had it pictured as filtering throughout my entire body. I didn't know anything about cancer then. I didn't know this was the most common type of breast cancer.

"I hung up the phone and said to Cyndi and Stanley, 'I guess this is it.' I thought it was the end of our life together because I didn't know of anyone who had survived cancer before. Then Cyndi started screaming, and Stanley's eyes filled with tears."

Later that night Harriette called her gynecologist from Judy's house to inform him her lump had turned out to be malignant. "He was shocked," Harriette said, "and I wanted to kill him. I knew I never wanted to see him again after that, and I didn't, except for a couple of times later, when I bumped into him in elevators.

"My husband cried on and off for days after we got the news. I was just numb and in shock. I could hardly believe it when the radiologist said my lump had probably been there for eight years. I'd hardly ever been sick before. The only problems I'd had were hormone-related migraines and heavy periods."

Harriette said the only way she thought to cope was by going back to work. "I returned three days after having the biopsy and kept my focus on my job and continued to exercise." Her modified radical mastectomy was scheduled for the following week, on a Friday, because she didn't want to miss any work.

When the time came for Harriette's mastectomy, she was never alone during the four days she stayed in the hospital. Family and friends surrounded her, and people telephoned and sent flowers. Judy visited and was there on Monday when Harriette got the lab test results from her surgeon. "The doctor said all of the thirteen axillary lymph nodes he removed were clear of cancer. That was the definitive factor. We knew my cancer hadn't spread."

It was good news. The infiltrating carcinoma had been a slow growing tumor, which originated in the milk ducts and had broken out into the fatty tissue of her breast. The mass had measured one centimeter. Harriette had learned that once the cancer cells leave the ducts, they can enter the bloodstream and travel to the lymphatic system or metastasize throughout the body. Eighty percent of all breast malignancies are infiltrating ductal carcinomas.

Harriette said her tumor had also been tested for estrogen receptors, the proteins to which estrogen attaches. Hers was positive. At the time the scientific community already knew estrogen hormones had a significant effect on breast tissue. Because the ovaries produced the estrogen that fed these kinds of cancers, one form of treatment was to remove them.

Harriette's surgeon, however, never mentioned removing her ovaries, something which would come to haunt her for the rest of her life. He didn't mention any other treatment for her although at the time Harriette began her journey with breast cancer there were clinical studies underway on hormonal treatments to block natural estrogen's effects. Tamoxifen was already being offered to postmenopausal women with advanced breast cancer and was being used in conjunction with chemotherapy for women whose cancer had spread to the lymph nodes. Being pre-menopausal, with clear nodes, Harriette didn't fit into this category.

Nevertheless, upon hearing that all of Harriette's nodes were clear, Judy flew from her friend's hospital room, elated. She would return later that evening with cake and champagne. "Everyone celebrated," Harriette said. "Ironically, though, even with so much support, I had no one who could really understand what I was going through. None of my friends had had breast cancer or knew anything about it. None of them knew anyone else who had had breast cancer either."

At the time it was not a topic people openly discussed, in spite of the fact that breast cancer had occurred since ancient times.[1] Most people didn't understand it, and a lot of people thought the woman herself had done something wrong to cause it. Even the medical community seemed baffled and uncomfortable that there was still no cure for breast cancer. It seemed to Harriette that there was no one she could confide in about her fears and no one who could warn her about what she was going to see when she took her bandages off.

"The day I was to leave the hospital, one of the nurses asked me if I wanted to see my incision," Harriette said. "It was the first time I'd been alone since I entered the hospital, and I was ready to look at it. Still, I felt the shock when I saw one side was totally flat and there was no nipple. It brought me back to the time when I was a kid and I was such a tomboy. I would only wear the bottoms to my bathing suit when I ran around on the beach." She remembered this with a sentimental laugh. "I never wanted to wear the tops."

Thinking back to those days made Harriette recall her grandfather. "He loved me so much," she said, "he would be horrified now to know what had happened to me. He was my best friend. He always made me feel like anything I did was okay. Being with him was not like at home where my mother was strict and there was never any positive feedback. My grandfather played dominos with me and Parcheesi. We would go to St. James Park and feed Blackie, a squirrel we named, who ate out of my hand. And then grandpa got sick. He had a couple of heart attacks, and my mother would leave me for hours, waiting in hospital lobbies, while she visited him. I remember feigning a limp so my mother would pay attention to me instead of leaving me in those lobbies. She took me to several doctors, and they took X-rays of my leg, but they couldn't find anything that was causing my limp. And then grandpa died. I was only nine, and I was devastated."

The day after hearing her nodes were all clear, the surgeon pulled the tubes that were no longer draining fluid from her incisions and told Harriette she could go home. "Stanley picked me up from the hospital," she said, "and on our way home I asked him to stop at the Hartwood Athletic Center. I told him I wanted to ride the bike. I wanted to make sure I was still okay.

"Stanley said, 'Are you *sure* you want to stop there?' I was sure, and when I rode the stationary bike, I felt excited and alive. Stanley kept saying, 'Slow down. Don't overdo it.' After the ride, I felt good, and I was confident I would beat the cancer.

"The next day, my chest muscles were so sore and tight I could only lift my left arm a little past waist level. No one had told me what to do about it, and no one had said anything about exercising. On my own, I lifted my arm and touched my fingertips to the kitchen wall. I made a mark where they reached and did that a few more times that day. I did it every day, walking my fingertips higher and higher, until I could lift my arm over my head."

Harriette took only a week off from work to recover and, during that time, decided to call the American Cancer Society. "I don't really know why I called them," she said, "but I was worried I wouldn't be able to swim. I just needed to see someone else who had been through this, someone who was still okay. A woman there told me about the Reach to Recovery program, and then she sent one of their volunteers to my house."

The Reach to Recovery volunteer had been through a similar experience with breast cancer. "She brought me brochures and pamphlets of resources for women undergoing treatment. She also brought a temporary prosthesis, a form stuffed with soft cotton that I could slip into my bra to help even out my appearance. Then she gave me a little handmade pillow to use to take pressure away from the sore places. She was the one who told me about lymphedema," Harriette added. "No doctor had ever explained that to me."

Lymphedema occurs sometimes after lymph nodes have been removed from the armpit and there are fewer nodes and channels left to drain the lymph fluid, which carries away byproducts of infection. Sometimes, the swelling is only slight or sometimes so severe it becomes chronic. It could happen soon after surgery or even years later.

"The volunteer warned me to be careful not to get cuts or burns or insect bites on that arm," Harriette said. "Anything like that could get infected and trigger lymphedema. She told me it was best to avoid lifting anything heavy with that arm and not to even carry a purse on that side."

Meeting with her Reach to Recovery volunteer had made a big difference for Harriette. She saw that someone else had made it through cancer and thought she could, too. Eventually, a year later, Harriette would take the Reach to Recovery training and become a volunteer herself.

CHAPTER 10

Prostheses in a Box

Coping in the aftermath of cancer surgery, if there is no more treatment, we look for closure so we can get on with our lives. With my sense of femininity left intact by my immediate breast reconstruction, any psychological doubts of that sort for me had been averted. The only reassurance I needed to help me on my way was the announcement from the oncologist that I didn't need chemotherapy. Harriette, however, had different issues, and she needed more.

At one centimeter, her tumor had been staged at I. Larger tumors were staged at II or III, and they required further treatment beyond surgery. Stage IV meant the cancer had already metastasized to some distant organ, and although there was treatment, there was no cure. Since all of Harriette's lymph nodes were clear, the standard protocol for a stage I tumor called for no more treatment and, therefore, she had no referral to an oncologist. Her surgeon had said, however, that because of where her tumor had been located, near her breastbone, she might want to talk to a radiation oncologist after her incisions healed. In the meantime there was nothing more for her to do.

"So I decided to exercise," Harriette told me. "I began riding the stationary bike every day at the Athletic Center, and then I started adding various exercises from my previous routine, minus the upper body weightlifting. I'd started the lifting only a short time before my cancer was discovered because I wanted to increase my strength to take care of Cyndi.

"Cyndi was still walking then, but she was very sick, suffering from avascular necrosis, a weakening of the bones, caused by the steroids she took to control her asthma. We always knew she would eventually be in a wheelchair and probably even bedridden some day, so I needed to be able to lift her. But besides that, I believed if I could get back into my former exercise routine, I could show myself and everybody else that nothing had been changed by the cancer. I thrived when things stayed the same."

Exercising again, Harriette felt herself healing physically. Her life seemed to be getting back into balance, yet she felt lopsided and uncomfortable with only one breast at a size 36DD. She felt self-conscious about her mastectomy. The Reach to Recovery volunteer had mentioned that Joslin's Department Store had a special section that fit women for artificial breast forms, so Harriette decided she would go there. It was time to do something about her problem.

"Being there took me back to when I used to go to a special store in the east, to get fitted for bras in my size. There were some flat-chested women in there who were being fitted for prostheses after their mastectomies. I remember thinking then how horrible it must have been for them. Now, it was *me* getting the prosthesis. I bought one and wore it to work, but I found it was bulky and heavy. It was too artificial, and I hated it.

"Luckily, though, I heard about Treva's, where they sell the 'Nearly Me' prostheses. So I went there and purchased one just before our wedding anniversary on November 4th. I was elated because this one had a nipple, and it was more natural than my first one. I wore it on our anniversary."

Harriette and Stanley celebrated at an elegant restaurant on top of Flagstaff Mountain. At six thousand feet above sea level, they dined on seafood and wine, overlooking the lights of Boulder and the University of Colorado campus. "I felt wonderful," she said.

Even with the "Nearly Me" prosthesis and the reassurance given to her by the Reach to Recovery volunteer that women can survive cancer, the fear of dying still haunted Harriette. So she sought out other means for support. "I joined the 'Back On the Move' swimming class at the YMCA. It was taught by a tiny, dynamic instructor named Gloria Kubel, who was well-known in the cancer community."

In Gloria's noonday class Harriette discovered all the women were post-mastectomy patients—many of them in poor physical condition. When she realized she was actually in fine shape compared to them, it didn't seem important anymore that she miss work to be in a swimming class. So she began swimming on her own at Hartwood. She took up tennis, too, and in time was back to her pre-surgery physical condition.

Despite feeling strong physically, a subtle feeling about the cancer still nagged her, and Harriette wondered whether radiation would benefit her. "I made an appointment for a consultation with a radiation oncologist," she said. "He said it was my choice whether to have radiation because my cancer had been a stage I. Since the tumor was less than two centimeters and I had no positive nodes, it was not standard practice."

Since her tumor had been located on the inner quadrant of her breast, though, microscopic cancer cells could have spread from the tumor to the chain of nodes along her breastbone, where they could be hiding under ribs. If this was the case, radiation would destroy them. Only a small percentage of tumors occurred on the inner quadrant, so it was not common to find positive nodes under the breastbone, but it was possible. More often, tumors were in the upper outer quadrant, where the lymph drains from the tumor into the armpit. If the cancer had started to spread, it would usually be found in the axillary nodes first.

Harriette had always thought radiation *gave* people cancer. In fact, during the early days of cancer treatment radiation *was* often damaging to nearby normal tissues, but since the 1960s doctors had used linear accelerators. The new machines are more precise at delivering charged particles onto the target. "The radiation oncologist reassured me that I had a ninety-five percent chance of the cancer never coming back if I had radiation," she said.

"So I went. It was scary the first time—the unknown always is." She remembered the simulation that was necessary on the first visit, when the radiotherapist took measurements and used a computer to plan the exact angle, shape, and depth of the rays to be emitted by the linear accelerator. Before she could begin treating the area on the middle of Harriette's chest, the therapist had to locate the specific spots that would receive the beam. She marked them with four tiny permanent tattoos. The beam would deliver a dose strong enough to kill cancer cells, without damaging Harriette's ribs or her heart, lungs, or skin.

For an hour Harriette lay very still while the radiotherapist measured and fed information into the computer. From these calculations she knew the exact dosage of rads and where to aim the beams every day for the next twenty-five days. After this first planning session, each succeeding treatment would only last a few minutes. "After she'd made all the calculations, she left me alone, lying on the table under the huge X-ray machine," Harriette said. "It seemed like a giant symbol of the cancer that could kill me. I just prayed it would work."

The next day and the next, Harriette broke from scheduling, updating doctors' curriculum vitas and answering the phones at Craig Hospital to go to Porter Hospital for her radiation treatment. "The treatments weren't so bad," Harriette said. "I got used to the noise of the machines after a while and hardly noticed any ill effects except for a little sunburn and fatigue. I think I was adjusting well to having lost a breast since I was used to working in a hospital where other people were adjusting to wheelchairs." After paralyzing accidents, many of those patients were left unable to walk.

In five weeks Harriette was finished with her radiation and all of her cancer treatment. Nevertheless, in January 1985, a few weeks after the radiation ended, Judy and the doctors Harriette worked with at Craig Hospital urged her to see an oncologist. "Just to be on the safe side," they said. Judy suggested her daughter's best friend's father, Dr. David Garfield.

"Dr. Garfield agreed with my surgeon, that there was no need for me to undergo chemotherapy, but he thought since I had such dense breast tissue, there was the chance that a mammogram might miss a possible tumor in my remaining breast. So instead of chemotherapy, he suggested I have a prophylactic mastectomy on the other breast. I wasn't resistant to it at all. Three months of anxiety and fear had taken a toll," she said. "I was wearing the prosthesis in a 36DD bra, and it was heavy. I was tired of being lopsided and uncomfortable with shoulder pain. I was paranoid about getting a new cancer in my other breast, and Stanley was worrying all the time, too. We agreed it was a good idea to do it, and I had the second surgery that same month. It was a huge relief."

She found it harder recovering from the second operation in spite of the fact that there was no additional incision under her arm. There had been no need to remove lymph nodes this time, but having a second surgery so soon after the first brought greater fatigue. "I went back to work and back exercising anyway. It just took me longer to recover. Then, my surgeon recommended I have double breast reconstruction. I knew right away I would never do it. I just didn't want to have to stop exercising to have more surgery."

When her parents came out from Whitestone, New York, in the summer, they too recommended she have the reconstruction. Harriette's mother had already been upset that a general surgeon and not a breast cancer specialist had done her daughter's surgery, and now the fact that her daughter had no breasts at all added to her discomfort. "What will people think?" she said, "This is a closet disease, and people aren't used to women with no breasts." She strongly urged Harriette to talk to a plastic surgeon.

Harriette consented just to please her mother, and they all went to the consultation. "We discussed the pros and cons of the surgery with the doctor," Harriette said. "And when he mentioned some of the possible complications, it just reaffirmed my conviction that it was not right for me. I'd heard too many horror stories from people who had suffered from infections and problems with the reconstruction. Stanley didn't care if I decided to do it or not. I asked my son, and he said he didn't care either."

To her parents' dismay, instead of the reconstruction, Harriette chose two "Nearly Me" prostheses from Treva's, in a size B, and wore them to work. "Later, I was self-conscious wearing the prostheses," Harriette admitted. "They were hot in the summer, and they shifted around under my clothes. They interfered with my biking." Soon, she stopped wearing them when she was at home. "I asked my son if he wanted me to wear them when his friends came over. He said he really didn't care."

Harriette had to keep the prostheses in a box when she wasn't wearing them, so they would hold their form. Since she was swimming and exercising daily and changing in locker rooms, she always had to carry the box with her. "I was shy about changing my clothes in front of other people. I'd cover myself with a towel because I thought everyone was looking at my chest. Then I realized many women are very small breasted and it didn't matter if I was flat-chested, so I eventually stopped using the prostheses altogether, which really upset my mother. I started lifting weights to build up my pectoral muscles instead. Besides, I wanted to get stronger to be able to lift Cyndi."

While Harriette was getting stronger and caring for Cyndi, she was putting her attention back onto her job at the hospital. At the same time, she started paying attention to the applications for Life Insurance Policies that were arriving in the mail. "They advertised 'quick physicals,'" Harriette said, "which meant that only blood tests and heart checkups were required. The ads made me think of what would happen to my family if I were to die from breast cancer, so I started responding to them." Over a period of time she accumulated eight different policies and then, assured that her family was provided for, put the cancer out of her mind.

With that worry aside and the prostheses permanently put to rest, Harriette could get on with her life. She decided to go back to school. Ultimately it took her six years to complete her degree, but she graduated with honors. The joy over her achievement and the lull from her cancer lasted, unfortunately, only one more year—until 1992.

CHAPTER 11

Mothers

I expected to learn soon the details of what happened in 1992, surrounding the return of Harriette's cancer; however, it would be several months before this would happen. In the meantime I was involved with other people and events, which took my mind off of Harriette for a while. They opened my eyes further to the realities of breast cancer.

First, there was the Day of Caring, an event held every spring near Mother's Day in Denver to promote breast cancer awareness and hope. Dr. McAleese suggested I go. "You'll love the fashion show," she said. "It's the best part." But it was the educational seminars that had the greatest impact on me. I came away from these sessions intensely affected by the fact that breast cancer wasn't a trivial matter. It was still indeed the same demon I thought it was the day I heard that breast cancer had stolen Linda Palmieri from us. The disease was continuing to take something valuable away—the lives of mothers.

When I arrived that morning, I was drawn to the opening ceremony by the sound of drums. Inside, I found a theater full of people who were celebrating "survival." A woman on stage with the drummers was directing everyone to make music with their hands. She was leading one part of the audience in a chant and directing another to clap in rhythm with the drums. I joined in with the third section, which was clapping in different rhythm. A fourth section sang a complementary chant. Our clapping and chanting continued until we'd transformed into a human symphony. With everyone's heartbeat aligned you could feel a powerful strength of oneness.

In the midst of the excitement a woman nearby caught my attention, and I recognized her striking smile. It was Kim Scott, a survivor I'd met only once before at the American Cancer Society. We connected again as if propelled by the magical vibrations. Kim was a Reach to Recovery volunteer who was reaching out to young survivors like herself. She was also interested in helping to increase awareness about issues unique to women in their twenties. Each of us thought we'd like to get together, so as the crowd began dispersing to various seminars, we promised we would soon.

It was funny that I next met up with Harriette on the way into the first seminar. When we sat down together, I was happy to see that Pat Grahn was there, too, seated across the crowded room. She was wearing the same fisherman's hat as when I'd met her at the ABCS. She caught sight of us and waved as the panel of breast cancer clinicians began introducing themselves. The panel presented medical information along with updates on research studies and clinical trials.

Even with as much reading as I'd done about breast cancer, much of what I heard sounded like a foreign language. I didn't know what immunotherapies were or molecular targets, nor did I understand when speakers talked about aromatase inhibitors and bisphophonates. By late afternoon I felt like I'd been immersed into a sea of drowning women, when many of them began raising their hands in a frenzy of questions for the panel. They were searching for answers. Unlike me, who believed I had been cured of breast cancer, they were in a battle for their lives.

Those taking tamoxifen wanted to know what else was there for them when their five years on the hormone were up. Was it safe to take estrogen after five years of tamoxifen? Their questions and personal stories brought the trauma of my cancer back to the forefront of my mind. Perhaps no one is ever "cured" of breast cancer, I thought. Like me, Harriette and Pat Grahn weren't raising their hands, but I wondered what they were thinking. I walked away from the meeting, stunned and overwhelmed by how much I had yet to learn.

The luncheon at the Day of Caring featured a fashion show moderated by our local television news anchor, Aimee Sporer, who I'd always thought was so beautiful and professional. The models, however, were not professionals. They were our peer survivors. Unashamed of their bodies altered by breast cancer, each one pranced proudly down the runway in new spring fashions. Aimee's commentary on each one included the model's diagnosis and treatment along with a description of her outfit. The audience celebrated each model with a hearty applause.

Contrary to Dr. McAleese's opinion, I didn't love this fashion show. I thought it was an exploitation of the women on stage, and it bothered me. By the next year, at my second Day of Caring, I would see that my attitude had changed, just like a lot of my ideas and thoughts about breast cancer would shift and change. I was truly able to celebrate each model and her recovery. But driving home after this first experience, my mind was busy, intently sorting through the events of the day. I had taken in every word of every moment, imprinting faces and committing stories to memory. I could hardly wait another twelve months until the next one. I wanted to learn more, but now I had to hustle home. There was housework to do and company coming for Mother's Day.

At home I was surprised to find the usual clutter in the garage had been cleaned up and straightened and the concrete swept. Inside the house looked different, too, from how I'd left it in the morning. Things had been picked up and put away. It was neat and clean. I wondered who had done this. "Did you do this?" I asked Jim.

He just smiled. I was shocked to discover that he'd stayed home from work all day to tidy the house for me. He hadn't done that in years. I knew it was because he wanted me to go with him to see the Colorado Rapids play that night. We had season tickets for all their soccer games. With no excuse that I had housework to do, I headed down the stairs to change my clothes.

I hadn't fully realized the impact of the day's events; it took a look into the bathroom mirror to trigger it. I saw myself first, but suddenly my face turned into those five hundred women at the Day of Caring, and I was overcome by the powerful image. We were each somebody's wife, somebody's mother, and somebody's sister. We had people who cared about us. We mattered. I mattered. And breast cancer was our threat.

Jim caught me crying in the bathroom and, worried, asked, "What's wrong? Did something bad happen?"

"No," I said. "Something good. Just leave me alone for a minute." I couldn't explain something I didn't quite understand myself. I cried more into a towel. The realization that I was valued felt enormous. The weight of it slipped into the towel, and soon it was over. With a splash of cold water on my face, I sensed a new life. I emerged from the bathroom announcing, "I'm ready to go to the soccer game." We had a good time there and a wonderful Mother's Day as well.

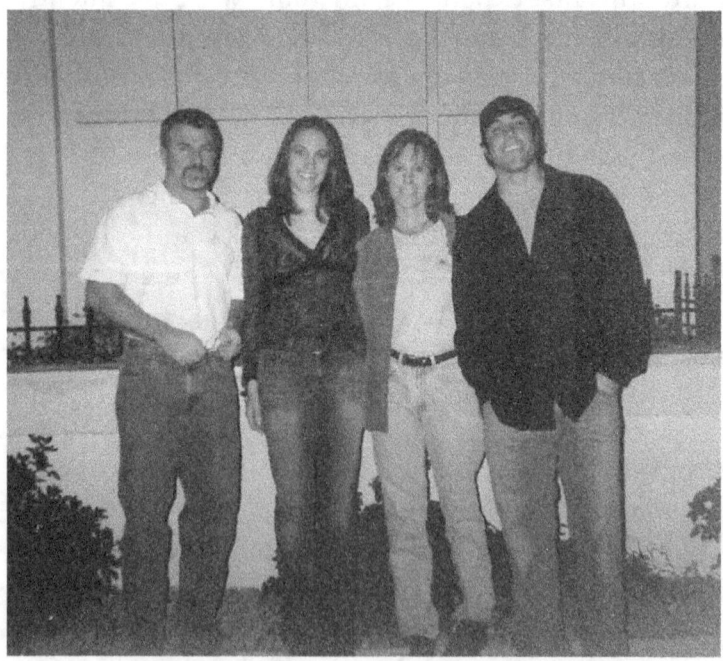

Jim, Heather, Diane, and Matt Chambers

Deep in the battle of "mothers against the demon" was Pat Grahn. I visited with her the following Monday. I was still reeling with emotion from the weekend as I drove to her house with the windows down. It was unusually hot for ten o'clock in the morning. For the fourteenth of May, it was too early in the season for such heat.

But I was eager to visit with Pat and was not worried about the heat. Since we'd met, she and I had talked a few times, and today I was going to her house for the first time. I, who had taken for granted that every woman had routine mammograms, would be surprised to learn that she had never had them. I would come to understand how a seventy-two-year-old woman had made her treatment decisions. I learned how she coped with the debilitating effects of her chemotherapy, and I would be reminded how precious mothers are to us.

Pat came to the door wearing a bubbly smile and a pale green turban, trimmed with white lace and embroidered flowers, around her bald head. She wore moccasins on her feet. Besides breast cancer, I noticed we had something else in common. "I have those same shoes," I said. They were comfortable Aerosols. "Only, I can't wear mine anymore because a mouse chewed up the back of one." She laughed, but I was mournful. I loved those shoes. Pat seemed energetic today. She said she was energetic now, two days before her next chemotherapy treatment, but wouldn't feel that way after.

She invited me to sit in a comfy blue easy chair in her living room, and she took a matching one next to mine. We chatted about me and my cancer at first, and then I asked her, "What kind of breast cancer did you have?"

Pat held a look of surprise. "I don't know," she said. "The doctor just said, 'You have cancer.'"

Pat told me she first noticed the lump in her right breast eight months before she saw her new primary care physician. She hadn't mentioned the lump to her previous doctor before he left her insurance plan because "He wouldn't have cared," she said. "Besides, I didn't think there was much reason for concern because the lump didn't hurt and there was no oozing from the nipple." Oozing, she thought, was the sign of cancer.

"I had just signed up for a machine quilting class that was to start in February and was on my way to see my primary care doctor, just to check on my diabetes."

In spite of her diabetes and her seventy-two years, she was in fairly good health. For a couple of years now she and her husband had been taking frequent walks, often three- or four-mile hikes around a park, not far from their home. Sometimes they drove up to the mountains to Estes Park to see the birds and the leaves while they walked.

"The walking keeps us fit," Pat said. "It's what helped me lose the 85 pounds that caused my diabetes in the first place. Since changing my diet and starting a serious walking routine, the diabetes has been well controlled without any medicine," she added satisfactorily. "I don't like taking medicines."

This was the first time Pat had seen this new doctor. "He was so nice," she said. "He made me feel comfortable, so I just casually asked him about my lump." The doctor felt the hard, anchored lump and looked worried. He patted her on the shoulder and said, "This might not be cancer, but I want it checked."

"Everything happened so fast after that," Pat said. "He left the room and called the surgeon right away. When he came back, he told me I was scheduled for a mammogram and an ultrasound and that he'd already made an appointment for me to see the surgeon. I'd never even had a mammogram before."

Pat wasn't alone. Even with increased awareness of breast cancer and passionate mammography campaigns, I found out that many women didn't routinely have them, some because they couldn't afford them or they didn't want to expose themselves to the radiation. Others feared the exam would be painful, and some women didn't get them simply because they feared what the X-ray might reveal.

Pat went to have her first one. "All of the ladies at the imaging center acted so kindly to me. The woman who did the mammogram was very gentle, and the technician who did the ultrasound apologized that the gel was so cold." Pat thought the technician was especially sensitive toward her. As she rubbed the transducer across the lump, she asked Pat, "Does this hurt?"

Afterward, when the technician told her to lie there for a few minutes while she stepped out of the room to find out whether there was anything more the doctor wanted, Pat suspected the woman had seen something on the screen but wasn't allowed to say what she thought it was. "The radiologist didn't say one way or the other as to what he found on the films, but I sensed some sympathy from the office lady who handed me my films." Pat was to take the films with her when she saw the surgeon the next day. "Their extra kindness gave me the clue I had cancer," Pat said.

Later, a surgeon looked over her films in his office. He examined her and said, "I think I know what it is. We don't even need to do a biopsy, but we will." He did a needle biopsy right then. The next day, when he called Pat, he said the report confirmed his suspicions. "It's malignant."

"I already knew," Pat continued. "I had never thought I would hear I had cancer. I was really scared. Then things started moving so quickly, I didn't have time to think much about it."

Pat wanted to do whatever the doctor thought she needed to save her life, and that was an immediate mastectomy. A lumpectomy was never discussed. "I never did get to the machine quilting class in February. I was scheduled to have a mastectomy the next week.

"My husband, Ray, was probably scared about it, too, but he didn't show it. He just said, 'We're gonna get through this.' It's been a 'we' thing from the start," she said. "I cried a lot at first, and then we called my daughter, to tell her about the surgery."

Pat coped with the apprehension of having to have a mastectomy by keeping busy. "I was sewing baby quilts up until the time for surgery," she said. "I got through the operation by convincing myself everything was going to be all right, and I didn't even feel too bad after the operation. I was walking around the hospital room, and my roommate, who was several years younger than me, remarked at how well I came through it."

Pat told me she saw an oncologist one month after she healed. "He told me I had eight lymph nodes with cancer and the surgeon removed nineteen. He said, 'You're going to need chemotherapy, and I suggest you get a port.' He told me my veins wouldn't last six months otherwise."

Pat couldn't remember whether her doctor ever mentioned what kind of breast cancer she had. She didn't know there were different kinds, and she didn't think to ask any questions about it. She didn't know what a port was either. The doctor just said it was something they would implant under the skin.

"The thought of having something foreign like a port in my body frightened me," Pat said. "I'd heard of people having trouble with things inside their body that weren't supposed to be there. But I knew the cancer was life threatening, and that scared me, too, so I would do what the doctor said."

Unfortunately, there was no test to find out whether any microscopic cancer cells had metastasized to other areas in her body. Doctors had to rely on statistics, which showed that women in a high-risk category, who had an invasive tumor over two centimeters and positive lymph nodes, had a greater chance of no further recurrences if they had a standard course of chemotherapy followed by radiation and hormonal therapies.

The chemotherapy would destroy malignant cells and all rapidly dividing cells. But there were different chemotherapy regimens, and they were chosen based on the woman's individual criteria. Pat's doctor decided on the drugs Adriamycin and Cytoxan for her, followed by Taxol (AC-T). It was a potent course of therapy that would take her six months to complete.

The drug combinations are more effective than using only one drug because each works in different ways to obliterate the cancer at various phases in a cell's life. Unfortunately, though, while the chemotherapy drugs were destroying Pat's malignant cells, they were also killing normal, healthy cells like hair follicles, blood cells, and those that line the mouth and digestive tract because these are also cells that divide rapidly. For this, her treatments would be spaced twenty-one days apart. The breaks would be long enough to give her body a rest, so her normal cells could repair themselves, but not long enough to give cancer cells time to begin proliferating again. And since not all of her cancer cells would be dividing at the same time, she would have to have the chemotherapy a number of times, spread over many weeks.

But first Pat needed a heart test. Since Adriamycin is toxic to cardiac muscle, a MUGA scan, short for Multiple Gated Acquisition, would show whether her heart could withstand the treatment. One in two hundred patients on this drug experiences cardiac side effects.[1] For the MUGA, a patient receives an injection of a radioactive substance, which attaches to red blood cells. Thirty minutes later, while she lies still on a narrow curved bed, a gamma camera rotates above her. The information from the camera is relayed to a computer screen, where the technician can view the heart muscle contracting. As the chambers pulse and pump the blood through, the amount of blood being squeezed from the left ventricle is measured. If 50–70 percent of the blood is ejected with each beat, the heart is functioning efficiently.

Beyond where she went for the MUGA, Pat could hardly remember having the heart test done. It was understandable, though. Memories often get lost in the whirlwind after a cancer diagnosis. They get filed in disarray in the mind, and it can take intense dredging to bring them up later. Doctors understand this about patients, too. They often say it's a good idea to bring someone along on appointments because after the patient hears the word "*cancer*," much of what comes later doesn't even register.

Apparently, though, Pat's heart was strong enough to withstand a course of Adriamycin, because here she was. After three months of chemotherapy, we learned that the mass in her breast had been an invasive lobular carcinoma. Lobular carcinomas were more often found in older, postmenopausal women. It usually meant that the other breast was also at risk for this cancer. The good news was that since lobular carcinomas have positive estrogen receptors, they're likely to respond to hormone treatment like tamoxifen, which inhibits breast cancer's growth. Pat would begin tamoxifen after chemotherapy and radiation.

"I went for outpatient surgery to have the port inserted. It's here above my left breast," she said, pulling the top of her blouse aside to show me the spot. It was purposely placed opposite her mastectomy side. When she woke up from the anesthesia, the small incision was numb, but under it was a bulge, shaped like a beer bottle lid, where the port lay beneath her skin. Invisible from the surface was a catheter, tunneled into the large vein in her neck.

Five days later, with the port still feeling tender, Pat rested in the lounge chair at the oncology clinic, waiting for her first chemotherapy treatment. If there were any microscopic cancer cells migrating in her bloodstream, the poisons in the bags hanging from the IV pole would kill them.

The oncology nurse manipulated a long clear tube from one bag and attached a needle at the other end. "She poked the needle into my port and gave me the first drug," Pat said. "It was a red medicine in two fat tubes. The nurse said, 'This is Adriamycin, and it will make your hair fall out in about fourteen days.'"

When the red tubes were empty, the nurse started the line from the clear bag, checking to see that it was dripping slowly and steadily to her satisfaction.

Pat had brought a book along to pass the time reading while the drugs dripped from the bags. "I hadn't read through two pages before the nurse came back to check on the drip and looked puzzled," Pat said. "She fiddled with the tube and said, 'This doesn't seem to be working. At this rate, you're going to be here for two days.' The nurse discovered my port was clogged and said the drug was going in much too slowly, if at all. She said we wouldn't be able to use my port, and so we had to use a vein."

The nurse located a vein in Pat's hand and took extra care when sliding the needle in. It was only the Cytoxan dripping now. If it had been Adriamycin and happened to leak from the vein, it could cause a severe burn on her skin. With added fluids, the veins can tolerate the drugs; however, if they became irritated and scarred, they couldn't be used for further treatments. "The IV in my hand was a little uncomfortable," Pat said, "but not too bad."

Ray drove her home after her chemotherapy treatment. Four hours later, the effect of the drugs became apparent when waves of nausea began to take over her last remaining sense of well-being. She lay curled up on her bed. When the vomiting started, her husband had to help her to the bathroom. "The vomiting continued throughout the night and for two more days, but we didn't call the doctor," Pat said. "I just kept thinking *it'll get better*. But after the third day of not being able to get up or keep anything down, I cried out to Ray, 'I don't want to live, if this is the way it's going to be.'" The intravenous anti-nausea medicine put into her IV with the cytotoxic drugs had not worked.

Finally, her worried husband called the doctor, who prescribed Zofran for her nausea. Zofran was a drug from the early 1990s. Though each pill cost between $20–25, it was a big improvement in treating the sickness others had endured over the years since chemotherapy had first been introduced. Patients of early chemotherapy had considered themselves guinea pigs while their doctors figured out which drugs and dosages to use; meanwhile, patients suffered with ineffective anti-nausea drugs that only clouded their minds and made them depressed.

"The little tablets dissolved on my tongue," Pat said. "They helped my nausea. The next day, I took more of them and was finally able to start eating a little Jell-O and applesauce. Ray was taking care of me, and he started fixing our breakfasts. He's been making them for us ever since, and he does the dishes now, too."

After she recovered from the first round of chemotherapy, Pat saw her surgeon again, fifteen days after he'd inserted the port. "I was upset and in tears," she said. "I told him I was having a lot of pain from the port and I didn't know if it was worth it. I asked him what would happen if I didn't do the chemotherapy. He said, 'You don't want to know. You've got to do this.'"

So, two days later, Ray and Pat were on their way to the hospital again, this time to see whether the port could be repaired. It was necessary to get it working in time for her second chemotherapy treatment. A different doctor would put in the new port in another outpatient surgery. Pat's regular surgeon shared his practice between Denver and another small town, where he happened to be working that day. But it was imperative that her treatment not be delayed, so his partner would stand in.

"I was sad and depressed that day," Pat remembered. "The first port hurt so much I dreaded going back for the second one, especially with another doctor." While she was asleep, he tried to repair the clogged port but was unsuccessful. He removed the port and sewed up the two-inch cut.

He then inserted the second port on her mastectomy side, higher up from where her breast had been. Normally, it was best not to have the port on the same side as the mastectomy, to reduce the chance of it interfering with the delivery of radiation, but in this case he had no other option. He made another one-inch incision at the side of her neck to ensure that the tube carrying the flow of medicine from the port emptied into the vein leading to the heart.

Now Pat had four incisions: a long one across the right side of her chest from the mastectomy, an accompanying cut under her right arm where the lymph nodes had been removed, and two on each side of her upper chest for the ports. The newer port site looked just like the first one had, like a bottle top placed under her skin. "It hurt to wear the car seatbelt over it," Pat recalled. "It stayed sore like that for over ten days."

Twenty-one days after the first treatment, it was time for the second. The Adriamycin had made her urine turn red for a few days and caused her hair to fall out just as she had been warned. This time, however, before the chemo, the nurse gave her two anti-nausea medications through the port, and Pat had her Zofran ready as well, to take at home. Knowing that the tablets would quickly dissolve on her tongue when she needed them gave her a little more comfort with taking a second treatment.

"I was working on my embroidery while the medicine dripped," Pat said, "and then I noticed the oncology nurse was struggling to find a good vein on a female patient nearby and a male patient was suffering from the same problem with his veins. Then the nurse said to me, 'Aren't you glad you have a port?' I hadn't considered myself lucky to have a port, but I did like having my hands free to sew.

"When the nurse asked me what I was sewing, I showed her the fabric squares I was working on, each with a different baby animal. I told her I didn't know what I was going to do with them. She admired my little deer and kitten and told me she was expecting a baby."

An hour and a half later, Pat went home and, with the increased doses of anti-nausea medicine, the side effects of the chemotherapy would not be as bad this time.

"I had only a little nausea, but the fatigue is awful," Pat said. After her third treatment, the side effects were the same. "I asked Ray, why do people take drugs if this is the way they make them feel? I did get sick on the third day, but mostly I have no energy.

"I'm a positive person," Pat continued, "always have been, but with this cancer, I have to work at it, to keep myself positive. Finding out I had cancer was a big shock. I do have my down times. Some people are not real kind with what they say. One friend said, 'Why do you wear those tacky hats? I wish you would wear the wig.' Well, I don't like wigs. I got one from the American Cancer Society. It's okay. I had it fixed by the beauty salon, but I prefer my hats, and they were nice in the winter because my head was cold."

Pat felt she had gotten a lot of support from her friends at church. "All I have to do is tell someone at church what I need, and it's here. My husband is wonderful, and I have my kids. I just keep on doing the same things I've always done, like make quilts for people, and I make these hats," she said as she patted hers.

"I have a good life," Pat said, gazing off toward her small dining room where her sewing fabrics lay folded on the table. "We don't see one of my sons and his wife much, but she called after my surgery, and she sent me a hat." Pat wanted to show me the hat. She pushed herself up from the easy chair and headed to the other room to get it. Her body rocked from side to side as she stepped to and from the bedroom. "For Mother's Day I got a box in the mail with this inside." She held up a wide-brimmed straw hat. It was white with a bright blue flower on the side. She removed her embroidered turban revealing her mostly bald head. Little clumps of thin white hair stuck out like those of a baby chick who had just pecked out of its shell. She put the hat on to model for me. "I wore it to church last Sunday," she added, smiling proudly.

"I noticed on TV that all of the people at the Kentucky Derby wore hats," Pat said. "Hats are the first things I look at now when I go into stores. I wasn't looking for a hat when I went into T.J. Maxx, but I bought a red one. I hate chemotherapy, but it's got to be, so I'm having fun with my hats."

"I like your hats," I said, noticing it was time for me to go. I told her I'd like to come back again sometime.

"I'd like that," she said.

As I drove from her house, I pictured her smiling in her white straw hat. Sometimes it took big things like breast cancer for us to see, in the little things, how much we are loved.

CHAPTER 12

Prophylactic Mastectomies

The next month I was still thinking about Pat, wondering whether she was doing all right with her chemotherapy, so I telephoned her. "I'm finished with Adriamycin and Cytoxan," she reported, like a college student announcing the end of finals week. "I'm on Taxol now. It still feels like poison, and I don't like it, but it's not as bad as Cytoxan." She was relieved to be entering the last stretch of her regimen.

"That's great," I told her. "You're almost done." I was glad she hadn't suffered with too many side effects. I still worried about her, though, since I'd read that the drugs affect the bone marrow. She could still be vulnerable to infections or get numbness in her hands and feet from the Taxol. But Taxol was recommended because it had been shown that it could significantly prolong survival over older chemotherapies.

The drug was originally made from the bark of the Pacific yew tree and was only offered at first to women in advanced-stage cancer. Since it was so effective, however, it had become more widely used.[1]

Pat said she was feeling strong, with no aches or pains, so this was reassuring. If her white cell count dropped too low, there were drugs like Neupogen to stimulate their growth and prevent infections. There were no drugs like this for my grandma when she suffered from infections and fatigue throughout her chemotherapy. I often wondered whether she might have lived longer had Taxol been available then. She might have suffered from its side effects, including allergic reactions, but there were drugs like Benadryl to prevent them. It seemed like a lot of drugs to have to take, and maybe they weren't too pleasant, but at least we had these options. I felt sorry for but grateful to those who had come before us, whose suffering helped us learn about all these drugs.

Pat told me on the phone she'd been making baby quilts since the last time I'd seen her. "A friend is going to have twins, so I wanted to make two similar quilts. I made one of them pink and the other one aqua. They're both bordered with yellow-checked fabric and lined in pink."

"I used to make quilts, too," I said with some nostalgia. "I'd love to see yours sometime." Pat apologized that she'd already given them away to her friend. I think she was hinting about putting her sewing away for a while, anyway, to start getting out more because she said, "I'm just looking forward to August when I'll be through with all of my treatment."

Since her diagnosis, she and Ray had curtailed almost all of their activities outside of the house because she hadn't been up to doing them. But Pat said she wanted me to come and visit again so we could listen to an audiotape of one of the sessions from the Day of Caring. A friend had loaned it to her after Pat missed the session. She had gotten too tired and had to go home. We decided we would listen to the tape on the day before her last treatment since she never felt too good for at least a week afterward.

Before we started the tape, Pat and I sat chatting in her living room. She rocked back and forth in the blue easy chair. She was not too tired today. "You look great," I told her. "Real chipper."

"Yes, I'm feeling good, but I've gained some weight right here." She laughed lightheartedly while patting her stomach.

"I understand chemo does that to you."

"Yes. It makes me feel funny, like I'm hungry, but I'm really not. I don't think I'm eating any more than usual. Tomorrow will be my last chemo, and then I'll be back to normal," she said, still rocking. "And my hair is growing back." She raised her hand to touch her head. She started laughing when she realized she'd forgotten to put her hat on that day. "I don't like to wear them in the house," she admitted. She put her head down and bent forward toward me so I could feel the fuzz that was growing back. "I didn't think it would ever come back. I thought I'd be wearing hats for the rest of my life."

It was nice to see Pat coming through the end of the tunnel of cancer treatment, wearing a smile and still focused on making other people happy. She told me the last time she had gone for her treatment she brought the baby quilt she made from the squares of embroidered baby animals. She had edged each square in bright blue and surrounded the whole quilt with a blue-checked flannel border. "It was hard to find the checked flannel," Pat said. "I had to make a special trip to the American Quilt Factory to find it. I gave the quilt to the pregnant oncology nurse as a surprise."

Pat's gesture toward her nurse made me think of how cancer professionals must feel about such gratitude from their patients. I was still thinking of that when Pat began showing me a couple of books she was reading. She held one in her lap and began to read aloud from another, a part where a woman had had a prophylactic mastectomy of her remaining breast after the removal of her first for cancer. "She did that to be *equal*," Pat exclaimed. "I can't imagine doing that."

"I can't imagine removing an undiseased breast either," I said, although I knew some women have felt like they have no choice.

Although it's a small percentage, some people carry the mutated breast cancer genes, BRCA1 and BRCA2. Women carrying these mutations are more susceptible to developing breast and ovarian cancers than the average person and at younger ages. Removing their breasts and ovaries before cancer has had a chance to develop seems like a life-saving measure, especially to those whose mothers and sisters have already developed cancer. I didn't know what I would do if I were in that situation. It didn't seem appropriate at the moment to share those thoughts with Pat. I just respected her feelings and recognized that everyone is different. We have to get through breast cancer in our own way.

Instead of debating this, I suggested that we start the tape. It was called "Your Diagnosis—Getting Through the First Year." On the tape, several women described their experience after diagnosis, the disruption to their lives and the whirlwind of emotions they had. One woman said she'd had times when her emotions flip-flopped every five minutes. Their stories brought back my own memories and a few tears, too. When I looked over at Pat, she was rocking softly in her easy chair. I couldn't speculate as to her thoughts, but I could see that, while we each chose different ways to cope to make ourselves feel whole and good about our bodies again, we were still very much the same.

CHAPTER 13

Broccoli Sprouts

Something women like to do is share and compare experiences with each other. After contracting breast cancer, we are no different. No matter our ages or what else we have in common, we like to talk about what happened to us. We like to see if we're better or worse off than our friends. Usually we find out we are not better or worse; we are just unique. There seems to be healing in this. Even though I was almost old enough to be her mother, Kim Scott and I wanted to get together. I visited her at her town-home a couple of months after the Day of Caring, as we had promised. Naturally, we talked about breast cancer.

We sat on the patio in her tiny backyard. There were no trees although the branches of the neighbor's young aspen hung over the fence into her yard. It was already over 80 degrees in the sun, but on Kim's patio the air was still fresh in the morning shade. Kim looked cool, dressed in a Danskin top and a long wrap-around skirt. As we sipped ice water, she began to tell her story.

She was only twenty-eight years old when she found a lump in her right breast. Young and single with hopes of marriage and children someday, she had much different issues facing her than older women do with breast cancer. Older women generally didn't worry about things like dating after breast surgery and trying to preserve their fertility, like Kim did. But she'd had one thing I considered an advantage, a sentinel node biopsy, which was still in the trial stages. The sentinel node biopsy is different than the traditional node-biopsy, during which surgeons remove a section of tissue from the axilla where thirty to sixty lymph nodes hide.

In the sentinel node biopsy, the surgeon injects a blue dye near the tumor and waits for the dye to penetrate the tissues. After she makes the incision, she can see where the blue dye has traveled and follow it to the first blue node, which is called the sentinel node. The surgeon removes the sentinel node and a few surrounding nodes and immediately sends the specimen to the pathologist. If the pathologist determines the nodes contain no cancer cells, then there's no need to remove any more tissue. It reduces the risk of problems later with swelling in the arm, which can happen when there are fewer nodes and vessels left to filter and drain away lymph fluid.

Kim told me about her biopsy and also what had been going on when she first discovered her lump. "It all happened so fast," she said. "It was the card hanging in my shower, the one with the pictures showing you how to do monthly self-exams and just a feeling I had, that made me do it."

Kim said she had looked at that card every day for eight years and had probably only done a self-exam about five times. "I was working for a design firm then and had just moved into a new home. It should have been a happy and exciting time, but I was overwhelmed. I had moved so many times before, and every time it had been hard for me. I was already living beyond my means, and suddenly things started going wrong with my car. It was falling apart, and I was scared to drive it. It had been stressful buying the house, and I was working so many hours. Then with the car problems, I just hadn't been able to deal with anything more at that time. But as I stood in the shower that day, something told me not to just *look* at that picture but to *do* the self-exam. That's when I found the lump."

Kim saw her doctor, who immediately ordered a mammogram. On the film there were no irregular dense white spots with extending streaks, nor any suspicious areas of tiny white clusters on the films. "My mammogram was clean," Kim said, "but sometimes things don't show up on X-ray through the dense tissue of younger women. My lump was palpable and solid, so the doctor said it needed to come out. Right then she went and made an appointment for me to see a surgeon."

Two days later Kim met the surgeon who would perform the lumpectomy. She had the lab test results. "The doctor said, 'Unfortunately, Kim, it's a cancer,' and suddenly I felt a surge of panic. But she had said '*a cancer*,' and I thought for a second maybe it was a kind that didn't kill, so I repeated the words like I hadn't heard them correctly, 'A *cancer?*'"

The surgeon answered *yes*. She believed it was an intraductal carcinoma, but they would only know for sure after surgery. "I asked her if intraductal carcinoma was bad and flooded her with more questions. She said mine was the most common kind of breast cancer and appeared to be less than two centimeters. However, in younger women, cancers tended to be very aggressive.

"Instantly, I felt compelled toward a mastectomy. I wanted to beat this cancer and the most radical treatment sounded like the sure path. But, the doctor said, 'At your age you might want to consider a lumpectomy, which will need to be followed by chemotherapy and five to six weeks of radiation.' She told me about the sentinel node biopsy and about a current study using hormone treatments I might be eligible for. But I was most worried about losing my hair, and I asked her if it was going to fall out. She answered by handing me a business card for a wig shop."

In the consultation the surgeon also covered the option of mastectomy and reconstruction. She passed Kim a photo album with pictures of actual reconstructed breasts and breasts after mastectomies. "I studied the photos, and when I turned to the pages of breasts with tattooed nipples, they just didn't look like something I wanted," Kim said. "I closed the photo album and said that maybe it would be better for me to see them in person or just do the lumpectomy."

In the days before surgery Kim's stomach was in knots. The knots persisted for days—to the point where she couldn't eat. Kim had recently become serious about her nutrition, and before this sudden change in events she'd been trying to lose weight. But now she *couldn't* eat, and the weight was dropping off. "I thought I was going to die, and I was only twenty-eight," Kim said.

She attributed her breast cancer to all the stress and junk food she'd eaten in her late teens and early twenties during a difficult adjustment time. "The doctor said my lump had probably been growing between four and seven years, and now I was afraid to eat anything. The only thing I ate was broccoli sprouts. I'd read somewhere that raw broccoli sprouts had high levels of antioxidants and phytochemicals—cancer-fighting compounds—so I bought several packages. I was practically shoveling them into my mouth by the fistful. They tasted awful, but I felt like I was doing something proactive, so I kept doing it." The sprouts were nearly all she ate for a week.

By the time Kim arrived at the hospital for surgery, she was ten pounds lighter from her diet of broccoli sprouts and worry. "I was worried about the blue dye and what it might reveal about my lymph nodes," Kim said.

Her surgeon didn't seem overly concerned, however. "She told me the dye doesn't necessarily mean there's cancer in the nodes, and anyway, she had a sophisticated European detecting device that was going to help her. I trusted her completely," Kim confided. "She was the chief resident."

As she was wheeled into the operating room, Kim spotted her surgeon dancing to jitterbug music at the scrub sink. "I knew then that everything was going to be all right," Kim said. Still, after the surgery, Kim's worry about her lymph nodes persisted. "I had to wait four days for the pathology report, and the thought of the cancer spreading was eating away at me. My surgeon had prescribed anti-anxiety medication and sleeping pills, but I was reluctant to use them."

Kim chose to deal with her anxiety without medication. When the news finally came, it was good. Thirteen nodes had been removed, and all of them were negative. "It was a big relief," Kim said. "I went back to work the following week, but still it was hard because some of my projects were multiple-page brochures that required clear focus and a lot of attention. I found that my work took me away from my cancer, and I *wanted* to be focusing on the cancer. I had decisions to make." Her oncologist would help with those decisions, but Kim would take an active role.

CHAPTER 14

The Quicker They Grow, the Quicker They Die

Whereas some of us choose to follow advice from our doctors without question, other women want to take more control over their treatment. And since there isn't a sure cure and one right way to treat cancer, we do what seems right for us. Concerned that her cancer was an aggressive one, Kim wanted to be sure she got the best treatment available. Before she spoke to an oncologist, she searched through bookstores and on the web for information on different treatment options.

What she learned about conventional treatment disturbed her. Radiation and chemotherapy could in themselves cause cancer. Yet in her research she also found statistics showing they significantly reduced the risk of a cancer recurring. Furthermore, the drugs supposedly worked better in premenopausal women like her. Kim grappled with the pros and cons of the treatment for a couple of weeks before her consultation with the oncologist.

On the day of her appointment she arrived looking disheveled yet resigned to taking the conventional treatment. "I sat across from the doctor already feeling uncomfortable because I hadn't showered that morning," Kim remembered. "I don't even know why I hadn't, because it wasn't like me. I was also uncomfortable with what he was saying. He said there was no cancer found in any of my lymph nodes, but the mass was almost two centimeters, and the Ki-67 was ninety percent. He said he'd never seen numbers that high before and wasn't even sure how to interpret them."

Ki-67 is a protein found in the tumor cells. A high number means that the cells are rapidly dividing, growing into new cancer cells. Usually, twenty to thirty percent was considered high, and Kim's numbers seemed to indicate an aggressive cancer.

"I thought this sounded ominous, and I said, 'Tell me something that will make me feel better about this.'"

His response was, "The quicker they divide and grow, the quicker they'll die, and the better the chemotherapy works. You're otherwise a healthy woman and should be able to tolerate the chemotherapy well."

If systemic therapy was begun without delay, it would destroy tiny errant cells that might have already traveled elsewhere in her body, cells which could lie dormant and become active later. He recommended Adriamycin and Cytoxan (AC) and then Taxol. "I wanted whatever would improve my odds, so I asked him if I could be treated even *more* aggressively than that. But my cancer was not estrogen receptor positive, and he said tamoxifen would have no added benefit for me." As Kim spoke now, she felt relieved about not having taken tamoxifen. "It would have shut down my ovaries," she said.

When Kim asked the oncologist about herbs and vitamins, he was reluctant to support their use because if vitamins stimulate cell growth, they might also stimulate the cancer cells. Vitamin E was his only concession.

With his advice, Kim began the chemotherapy treatments, but she also, contrary to his recommendation, made an appointment to see a specialist in herbs and nutrition.

A couple of days later she met with a naturopathic consultant, whom she found through the phone book. After assessing her concerns, the consultant suggested a diet and an extensive program of supplements.

"I was swallowing over one hundred pills a day, including 10,000 mg of vitamin C," Kim said. "I took milk thistle for liver support and L-glutamine for intestinal support. I took vitamin B and astragalus root, shiitake, and ashwagandha." For its anti-tumor effects, she downed tablespoons of unprocessed royal jelly and raw honey.

Kim believed the supplements would help rebuild cells destroyed by the chemotherapy and radiation. She took handfuls of them at a time and even carried them in little plastic bags to work. She started eating salmon and other fish, too, for their omega-3 fatty acids because they are believed to block tumor growth.

"I felt in control this way, and I believed I was going to do this for the rest of my life. It was how I could deal with my cancer. My parents were supportive, but I was changing my lifestyle on my own."

CHAPTER 15

No Mention of Reconstruction

———————◆———————

Even with little in common besides our breast cancer, I considered Kim, Harriette, and Pat my friends now, and I kept in touch with each of them often, either by phone or in person. If one of us suddenly had a recurrence, it seemed important that we be there for one another. Until there was a cure for breast cancer, we were all in this boat together. We were a sisterhood floating downstream, rooting for each other's full recovery.

I knew Pat was undergoing radiation in September, and I was concerned that it might be making her sick, so I called to see how she was doing. She wasn't home the morning I called, so I tried again the next morning. My concern was relieved when she answered. "I was getting my radiation yesterday," she told me. "Normally, I'm getting it every day at this time, but the machine's not working today. They said sometimes the machine doesn't work and I'll have to make up the days at the end." It was her second week, and she sounded upbeat.

Pat had finished all of the cycles of chemotherapy and had waited a week before starting tamoxifen and radiation. "I'm being cooked, and I'm halfway through," she said half-heartedly. The high-energy gamma waves were penetrating her skin on a mission to destroy stray malignant cells. At day fourteen, she was knocking off days from the required total of twenty-five.

Since I never had it, I wondered what getting radiation was like. "How do they do it?" I asked.

"Well, they're radiating the lymph nodes under my collarbone and under my right arm, so I have to lie perfectly still while the machine moves around me," Pat said. "It shoots radiation from three different angles, one straight, one from the left, and one from the right. I have to hold my arm up for my right side. I try to count how many seconds it lasts, but I get lost."

Pat said she had ten tiny dots permanently tattooed onto her chest showing where they had carefully calculated and mapped out the area. The tattoos had stung when she got them, but now they easily served as markers for the daily doses of radiation. "I was worried about leaving the port in during my radiation, but the doctor said it would be all right, as long as it was flushed out every month." The port would remain there for several more years, in case she was to need it again.

"I was worried you might be feeling sick," I said.

"No, I'm not, except for a little dry cough once in a while and feeling a little dizzy. The dizziness kept me from going to church on Sunday. I'm supposed to be drinking more water for that. And I can't wear a bra because my skin is so tender. It's only a little pink, though. There are no blisters."

I told her I was glad it hadn't been too bad for her. Quietly, I was relieved it hadn't burnt her skin black like I imagined it might, when I remembered Grandma. It would not be until nearly a year after Pat told me this that I became enlightened about radiation. After much research I finally came to understand that I'd been carrying the wrong assumption about radiation. What I'd seen on Grandma's chest were the black scabs of her dying skin tumors, not burned skin. Grandma's skin would have healed, I learned, had she lived.

But the radiation did cause Pat some fatigue. "I can only do one or two of the house chores each day. If I do the washing, I can't do anything more. If I clean the bathroom, I'm zapped." Other times, she said she found herself getting teary and didn't know why.

I wasn't sure how to help Pat, but I thought a visit might help keep her spirits up, so I asked whether I could see her. She said yes, and a week later I arrived at her home. As I'd been worried about her coming down with an infection, I found out she *had* suffered one episode. Pat gleefully showed me a number of her hats, in prints and plaids, solids and stripes, along with one large brimmed straw hat. I was busy admiring them when she divulged that she'd been sick.

"It began four days after I started taking tamoxifen," she said. "I felt so bad on Sunday that I took one of the pain pills I had left over from my mastectomy surgery."

Three days later, she said, she was still feeling poor with fever when she noticed some red blotches all over her left leg. "I blamed the tamoxifen at first. Then, I thought the pain pill must have been bad, too—old or something."

The red blotches had itched and spread to both of her legs until they became fiery red from her knees on down. Her legs swelled until it was too painful for her to walk, even to the bathroom. Ray had to help her. "I thought the cancer was spreading and I was going to lose my legs," she said. She bought some cream for the itching and refused to scratch her legs because she knew she wouldn't be able to stop once she started.

"The doctor said it was an allergic reaction and told me to take Benadryl. Later, when I went in to see him about the swelling, he said it was 'cellulitis,' an infection, and prescribed antibiotics. My friend's husband died from cancer, and she told me that my infection was probably from the chemotherapy. It lowers your resistance," Pat told me.

Whereas I'd learned about the risk of infection from books, Pat had learned it the hard way, by experiencing it herself. I commiserated with her for a while, and then she said even though she'd been sick, she had sewn another baby quilt with a big blue teddy bear appliquéd in the middle.

"Could I see it?" I asked.

"I already gave it away," she laughed. She'd given it to another church friend who was pregnant. Sadly, the friend's baby was later stillborn, and the teddy bear quilt had been used at the memorial service instead. It had covered the table for a "Precious Moments" urn, which held the baby's ashes.

I wasn't able to see Pat again until December, after she proudly told me she'd finished all of her treatment. I was thrilled. She seemed to have made it through with a total adjustment. "I'm wearing my prosthesis now," she said. She had worn it in a new comfortable bra she'd bought from Nordstrom's, even though it had been expensive. Although her husband didn't care whether she wore it or not, Pat did wear it whenever she went out. It didn't hurt her anymore like it had when it rubbed against her radiated skin. And Pat and Ray were getting out more. Recently, they had gone to hear the Sweet Adelines' Christmas concert.

It felt good to see Pat active again and so happy with her new prosthesis. Still, I wondered whether she had considered reconstruction. I was pleased with the results of mine and thought maybe she would like reconstruction, too. When I asked her whether she had thought about it, Pat said not one doctor had mentioned it. "All they do is take my blood," she said. "Every time I go there, they take blood. My oncologist says some doctors will tell you you're cancer free, but there's really no way to tell that. Cancer is invisible."

It seemed she was not interested in talking about breast reconstruction. She was more interested in getting on with living. "I'm just debating whether to put up a Christmas tree since it would only be for just Ray and me. Years ago we used to go to tree farms in LaSalle to cut our own tree," she remembered. "Now we have an artificial tree, which we spent a fortune on."

Pat admitted she didn't really feel like doing any decorating for the holidays, but she'd felt good enough to get out to a beauty shop for her first haircut since it all fell out. "It's growing back in all different lengths, and I didn't know what to do with it," she laughed.

Equally positive, Pat was attending church again. She was the teacher for the Cradle Row class—the toddlers. "I'm rusty, though," she said. "I was out for a year, and the songs aren't coming back to me too quickly." Pat had researched her techniques and was proud of her teaching methods with the little ones. She used songs and toys to stimulate their keen senses. She started to sing one for me in a lovely full voice, "Oh what a beautiful morning, oh what a beautiful day."

At the end of our visit, I said I'd like to come again in a few months. Pat smiled and said she'd like that. I left feeling good about her prognosis yet still pondering why no one had mentioned reconstruction to her. Was it her age that made doctors automatically assume that she wouldn't be interested, or was there some medical reason that she wasn't a candidate for it? Perhaps they assumed that a silicone breast form would be all she'd need to preserve her sense of femininity. Reconstruction had been offered to me immediately, and outside of the initial adjustments, I'd been delighted with the results. Pat seemed to have no issue on the subject, though, just an easy acceptance of herself, and I respected her for that. I wouldn't make it an issue either.

CHAPTER 16

Is It Medicine or Is It Art?

In my old life—life before breast cancer, when I wasn't busy with the kids and their gymnastics and soccer activities—I put most of my energy into interpreting and my professional interpreter organization. Since Jim worked long hours in his construction business, I had time to volunteer as the secretary for the organization for many years. Later, I became the workshop chairperson and then the Silent Weekend co-coordinator for ten more years. My friends then were other soccer moms or interpreters.

Now Heather and Matthew were away at college. Jim was still occupied building houses, but I was drawn more to my writing groups and to the sisterhood of breast cancer survivors. I gave up paying interpreting assignments so I could write, and I chose driving long distances to spend time with survivors over going to meetings with interpreters. As interpreters, it seemed we were always busy trying to make everything perfect. Survivors already knew you couldn't make anything perfect. Survivors were busy celebrating life. So, on a Saturday in July, instead of going to an interpreter meeting, I gathered with the women at the Association of Breast Cancer Survivors.

Our speaker that day was a certified strength and conditioning specialist, who was demonstrating how to use a giant bouncy ball in various ways to improve our fitness. "Unfortunately, exercise can improve every illness except cancer," he said, "but being as fit as possible will help you *feel* better."

He had several different sized balls for us to try, and Harriette and I took turns with one. With the giant ball pressed between the wall and my backside, I executed a few leg squats, rolling the ball down the wall. "The ball makes it feel easy," I said to her. After she tried it, we did a few more exercises. We agreed we liked it, and I thought I might buy one for myself. But Harriette said she didn't have room in her house for a ball that size. "My house is tiny," she said. "Why don't you come over and see it? You can meet my daughter, Cyndi, and see her art work."

Cyndi's projects were multimedia abstracts, which she created out of the medical supplies the doctors used for her treatments. Some were three-dimensional, and each one had a story. "It's hard to explain them to you," Harriette said. "You'll have to see them for yourself. You'll recognize our house easily; it's the one with the wheelchair ramp in front."

Two and a half weeks later, I rang the bell to her house. Harriette opened the door, smiled wide when she saw it was me, and yelled behind her, "Diane's here. I told you she's always on time." She led me into the living room, where the walls were heavily decorated with artwork. An electric stair transporter lined a narrow staircase directly across from the front entry. The small rooms of the house were crowded with furniture, an oxygen tank, and other medical equipment. Art projects and supplies were piled high in numerous places, including the dining room and kitchen tables. It was hard to distinguish which supplies were for Cyndi's medical condition and which were for her art projects.

Peeking around the corner of a display case into the kitchen, I glimpsed a young woman in a wheelchair. Her short black hair was pulled away from her face by a beaded headband. Her thin legs dangled from the seat like a floppy doll. "I'm coming, I'm coming," she called.

"You must be Cyndi," I remarked. "Your mom's been bragging about you. Did you do this?" I asked, pointing to a framed pencil drawing of a little girl hanging on the wall.

"Yes, that's my cousin, Heather, when she was four years old."

Cyndi had used seventeen different pencils on the portrait, which won an award in an international competition in 1986. Next to it was a portrait of Heather's brother when he was four years old. Cyndi drew him holding a telephone receiver to his ear. "He's all grown up now and, still, he always has the phone to his ear," she said.

I turned to the opposite wall to look at the three-dimensional abstracts behind the dining room table. "Tell me about these." They were made from plaster gauze, dipped into watercolor, and then preserved with glue coatings and shellac.

"It's called 'Super Nova,'" Cyndi explained. "I did those in 1988 and 1989. The colors represent my feelings—red for heat, pain, and fever, black for depressed or dying. The other is called 'Sombrero.' It's people dancing. Everyone has different interpretations of my art. My cardiologist has bought several pieces. I had one called 'Genesis' that was as big as this table." She gestured toward the dining room table, piled with stuff. "I had to lie on top of it to work on it. It had an egg and little sperms, all made from plaster gauze."

Cyndi had developed her art skills by taking a home study class and had been producing her creations for twenty years. Each one of the twenty or so displayed around the living room and up the stairwell had a title and a theme.

"'Incognito' is the name of this one. It's me as a boy. He wears a pouch. Because I feel trapped and can't escape, I put all of my feelings into the pouch. And because I tend to hide my feelings, I disguised myself as this boy."

Cyndi's little dog jumped into her lap. "I always wanted a dog, but since I have so many allergies, I couldn't have one. Then, when Mom got sick, we thought a dog would be a good companion for me, so first I had to get tested to see if I could have one." When the tests came out okay and the doctors said she could have a dog, Cyndi and her mom hurried over to the Washington Street Kennel to adopt one.

Harriette chimed in to our conversation. "We looked at various dogs, and she ended up choosing the ugliest one. She fell in love with him."

Cyndi defended her choice. "I picked him because he put his paws over his face when I picked him up from the cage. When he did that, I knew he was the one for me. I named him Garfield after Mom's doctor. He was our first dog. He was a Brussels griffon, a wonderful dog, who did tricks. Then he got sick with allergies and cancer, just like Mom and me. We had him for eight and a half years, and now we have these two, a cock-a-poo and an affenpinscher."

Cyndi showed me the rest of her artwork, including a collage she'd made with paper cut from colostomy stencils and an abstract made with melted plastic. The last one she showed me was created using egg tempura. "Because I'm allergic to oils," she said. She explained that she'd taught herself to draw from anatomy books and pointed out one picture she had drawn of a cowboy with one side of his face distinctly more aged than the other. "I made it like that because people don't realize that most of us age faster on our left sides."

Toward the end of the art tour, Cyndi started breathing harder and wincing from muscle spasms. She asked her mother to get her methadone. "I'm no longer able to do my artwork," Cyndi said. "I drop things, and with these spasms I ruin my work. Paper clay is the only thing I can work with right now." It wasn't a complaint of feeling sorry for herself; it was only a statement of how things were.

Cyndi's long-term use of steroids to control her asthma had caused the painful necrotic bones that plagued her now at the age of thirty-six. The condition was irreversible. She was taking the methadone four times a day for the pain. With her mild dysphagia (trouble swallowing), they had to put the pills in applesauce to make them easier to swallow. Sometimes she took up to 126 pills a day, so they put them together into capsules so there would be fewer of them to swallow. As I watched her struggle, I wondered how she would survive if anything happened to Harriette.

For the rest of the visit, the three of us sat on their back deck, lunching on salad and chocolate cookies. An umbrella provided shade from the intense sun as we chatted about my family and the book I was writing about Bert, my elderly deaf-blind student. Cyndi and Harriette were curious about him. They wanted to know how I used sign language with him when he couldn't see it.

"He feels my hand-shapes with his hands," I explained. Harriette wanted to know more, but unfortunately it was time for me to go. "I have an interpreting assignment I need to get to."

"At least take a cookie with you," she said, handing me one. "They're fat free." I ate the chocolate cookie in the car, delighted that I had come. I had found Cyndi interesting and pleasant. I had gained a new perspective about life forces that keep people pushing forward. Now I understood what kept Harriette going. It was her daughter.

CHAPTER 17

Chemo, It's My Lifeline

I'd just finished eating my pancakes when Harriette showed up a little late for our brunch at the Perkins restaurant, on September 4, 2001. She wasn't always perfectly on time, but she never canceled either, even when she was facing overwhelming challenges, which seemed to be the case every day. I'd come to see that Harriette didn't let anything slow her down. She seemed to stand out among the ordinary.

Apparently, other people had noticed that about her, too—long before I met her. She'd been profiled earlier that year in *MAMM* magazine—a cutting-edge publication on breast and reproductive cancers that was launched in 1997. When a representative from *New York Magazine* had called the Colorado Breast Cancer Coalition state coordinator, Anne Weiher, looking for an interesting story on a Colorado breast cancer survivor, Anne could have chosen a number of women, but she immediately thought of Harriette, who was one of the coalition's members. After Harriette agreed to be interviewed, a reporter and photographer flew out to Denver to spend an afternoon with her.

I'd never heard of *MAMM* until I met Harriette. When I read the article in the May 2001 issue, I saw that the reporter, Laura Bend, had captured Harriette's essence perfectly by using Harriette's own voice: "I was recently with a group of friends and each person listed three inanimate objects they would take with them if they were escaping a fire. Most of them said things like passports, pictures, photo albums, that kind of thing. For me, the first thing to pop into mind was just obvious—my Day-Timer."

The article was titled "Dogged Determination."

Now, Harriette apologized for being late as she slid into the booth. She'd already had a morning full of challenges. "I lost my pager this morning and was looking all over for it. I need it so my family can get a hold of me. Then, I got tied up on the phone with the insurance company. They're threatening to cancel my husband's insurance because he's had two accidents. I was supposed to go to a meeting with legislators today for the breast cancer campaign, but I've got an abscessed tooth that's killing me. No one's had a surgeon on call this weekend, and I've had to wait three days with this pain. Finally, I'm on antibiotics, but now I can't find a doctor for Cyndi. No one wants to take Medicare and Medicaid patients anymore. She needs some teeth pulled. I'm hoping the Dentistry for the Handicapped program will help pay for it. I don't know what we're going to do."

I was aware of the Medicare problem. Many doctors were refusing to accept new Medicare patients because the reimbursement by the government was not keeping up with the physician's cost to treat these patients, who often required a lot of their time.

"Maybe this isn't the best time for us to get together," I said. "It sounds like you have important things to take care of today."

"No, I want to be here. I want to do this." She calmed down and smiled.

"Okay, if you're sure," I said, taking the last sip of my coffee. I was hoping she would stay. I wanted to be with her. I wanted to learn about the chemotherapy she'd been on for years. I asked her to tell me about it.

"I go to the Rocky Mountain Cancer Center every other Friday for IV treatments. Last June, after I'd been on chemo for nine years, I started having pain in my hips and in my right buttock. I thought it was arthritis, so I went to see an orthopedist. He asked, 'Who's your oncologist?' He knew the pain was coming from my metastatic cancer. He figured I had some tumors pressing on a nerve, and he was right. We found out my cancer had become active again. I was disappointed to find out, but I wasn't surprised. I knew that after a while tumors become resistant to the drugs. I'm lucky, though; the tumors are there, but they're not growing. They haven't become resistant. I have dumb tumors," she laughed proudly, as if she had grown familiar and comfortable with her cancer.

Harriette had been getting intravenous chemotherapy every other week since 1992. "I don't hate chemotherapy like some people do," she said. "It's my life line! They told me I would be on chemotherapy for the rest of my life, and I just got used to it. I don't like it, though, when the doctors change things. I tell them, 'It's working, leave me alone.'" She laughed again. "Some people hate it when their treatment stops because they're scared when there's nothing else to lean on."

Her chemo gave her a sense of security. I would come to see that we all needed something to lean on. Without drugs to lean on, we turn to friends—to the sisterhood. When we finished our lunch at Perkins, Harriette invited me to come with her the next time she went for her treatment. "I'd like to," I said.

CHAPTER 18

The Cancer Center

The Cancer Center is a place most people don't like to think about. I think it horrifies them to imagine what they might see in there. Before I had melanoma I used to be like that. When I saw the sign in the hospital that said Cancer Center, I felt creepy walking past it. It scared me that cancer might happen to me someday and I would have to go there. I wondered why anyone would want to work at the Cancer Center.

People who have cancer prefer not to have to go to the Cancer Center either, but they go, and we think they're heroes because they do. But they don't think of themselves as heroes. They go there because they desperately want to get well, and they've opted to take the risk that the side effects of cancer treatment will be worth the benefits. And all the kind souls who work there desire for that, too, because they very much want to help patients get well.

I wasn't afraid to go near the Cancer Center anymore. I wanted to see it and to find out what they do in there. Since the people there had kept Harriette living this long, I figured it must be a good place. Besides, I wanted to be with Harriette. Who knew, some day I might need to be at the Cancer Center, and I might like somebody to be with me.

So on September 21st I met up with her at the Rocky Mountain Cancer Center near downtown Denver. Our city is famous for its Indian summer days, and this was a picture perfect one, though a little too much on the warm side. The temperature was in the high eighties—too hot to wear stockings with my jumper and cotton T-shirt—so I opted for bare legs and sandals. It was cool inside the building, though, and I found Harriette in one of the small treatment rooms. She was expecting me.

Right away, I noticed she was friendly with the medical assistants who passed in and out of the room. It seemed everyone knew her. She chatted with the oncology nurse—who was pushing a needle into the Infusaport in Harriette's chest—about a bike trip she had done with her son Jeff over the weekend. Harriette introduced me to the nurse. I watched her draw some blood from the needle, and then I asked her what the blood was for.

"We need to check her levels of INR (international normal rate) and her Prothrombin time," the nurse said. It was the measurement of her blood plasma clotting time because the Coumadin pill Harriette took every night thinned her blood. It prevented the blood clots or pulmonary embolisms, which are potential risks of cancer. They had to monitor her blood carefully so it didn't get too thin, to where she could have internal bleeding.

"When I have major dental work done, I have to go off of the blood thinners," Harriette told me, "or I could have a problem with bleeding. But what Harriette really wanted to talk about was the weekend she'd just had with Jeff. "We rented a tandem in Glenwood," Harriette told the nurse. "I didn't like it. My son had all the control, and I kept yelling, *brake*! He'd say, 'Cool it, Mom!' He had to work harder than I since he was the one in front."

The nurse laughed while another one began to hook up the line for Harriette's Aredia. I watched her fasten the needle in the port with tape before she pushed a syringe full of Leucovorin into the IV tube. Leucovorin is a vitamin derivative of folic acid that works as a binding agent to the chemotherapy drug, 5-fluorouracil, known as 5-FU. It helped it work better. Five hundred mg of 5-FU followed the Leucovorin, and both drugs went through the syringe in less than five minutes.

The first nurse fiddled with the pump that was supposed to begin dripping the clear bag of Aredia through the IV. "Darn it," she complained, "I don't like these pumps." All the while, Harriette continued talking about the bike ride and about registering for the upcoming Race for the Cure. Harriette said she was looking forward to the race in October. Her drive amazed me.

Whereas she came here twice per month for chemotherapy, Harriette only needed Aredia once a month. On those days she sat here in a private room for almost three hours. From a soft leather chair she could face the big picture window and look out at the huge shade trees and homes of Capitol Hill. Today, she stretched out in the chair with her feet up. The bag of Aredia hung ready from an IV pole. It would take two hours to empty, so we had plenty of time to visit. Mostly, Harriette talked, and I listened.

"I went to workout for an hour this morning, though I didn't feel like it," she said. "I knew I would be too tired to do it after the chemo. Besides, in the pool I can really get away from everything. There are no pagers, no phones." She said the chemo always wiped her out for a few days and made her nauseous if she didn't eat. Harriette said that over time she had learned to plan her activities around the inevitable fatigue that followed her treatment, and for that reason did her bike trips with her son on her "off" weeks.

"I got here early today so this could drip in slowly," she said. "If it goes in too fast, I get sick." She was referring to the Aredia, which I'd learned was a bisphosphonate that worked at preventing bone pain and curbing her bone tumors' growth, though it was harsh on her kidneys. Harriette told me she had to drink a lot of water after these treatments to protect them. But it was easy for her. Since the very beginning of her chemotherapy, she'd been drinking twelve glasses of water a day. She learned the importance of drinking plenty of water from biking. "I used to become light-headed and nauseous from dehydration. Now, I'm drinking water all day out of habit, not just on chemotherapy days."

Harriette knew I was interested in learning everything I could about cancer and chemotherapy, so like a teacher she patiently explained things to me and even spelled words that I couldn't quite make out because of her New York accent. I always found the facts interesting. "I used to get 750 mg of Leucovorin with the

5-FU," she continued. "It cost $1,500. But then, in 1996, they figured out I didn't need that much, and now I get only 50 mg. The 5-FU is cheap in comparison to Leucovorin."

Harriette reflected on when she'd had her first port inserted, when she insisted on being awake for the outpatient surgery, because she wanted to go back to work and didn't want to feel groggy all day. "I remember they had trouble getting it in. Then one day, seven years later, when I was getting my chemotherapy, the port just blew. It clogged up or something, and the medicine couldn't go in. It went all over me instead."

She was laughing about it now, but I could see it wasn't funny at the time. "The nurses had tried to unclog the port, but it didn't work. I had to go get an X-ray right away, so they could see what had happened. They told me it was going to have to be replaced. I had to take my chemotherapy through a vein that day, and for several days after I worried that I was going to have to pay out-of-pocket for the port replacement. I'd just joined a new HMO, and I wasn't sure they would cover it.

"Luckily, the HMO did pay for it. Now I have this new port in the same place as my old one. I've had it for two years. The doctor was relieved he got it back into the same spot. It wouldn't have been good to put it on the side where my lymph nodes are gone."

"That's good," I said, relieved.

Harriette admitted she felt tired today. She had been to two medical appointments with her daughter already. "Cyndi has a personal care provider five days a week for a couple of hours, but that person can't drive her to appointments, so Cyndi always wants me to do it. It took up most of today because Cyndi's so slow. She has an ileostomy, and her hygiene takes a lot of time."

Harriette told me she'd been so busy and tired that something scary had happened to her while she was driving. "I fell asleep at the wheel last night at 10:30. I woke up, suddenly, because someone behind me honked. I didn't know where I was at first." Fortunately, she had been stopped at a red light when she nodded off.

I could see she was tired. She told me she usually got a lot done here while she received her treatments. Sometimes she napped. I didn't want to infringe on that time today if she wanted to nap, so I kept our visit short. I told her I had to go, but I was pleased when she invited me to come back again the next time.

On November 16th I was sitting in the lobby at the Cancer Center waiting for Harriette. At two o'clock in the afternoon nearly all twenty seats in the waiting room were full. The place was bustling. With five medical oncologists and four hematologists on staff, it was not surprising. I remembered Harriette commenting once that she thought this center was more impersonal than the old place she'd been to on Franklin Street, where all the patients used to get their treatment in one big room together. "Now, there are many private rooms for the people who don't feel good," she'd said.

Today, an elderly couple slept leaning against one another in a shared loveseat. A tall, very thin young woman walked slowly from the treatment rooms, alongside an aide. She wore a blue bandana over her bald head and looked like her clothes had recently become a couple of sizes too big for her. Another woman, about forty-five, wore nothing over her hairless head. She sat reading a journal from the rack on the wall that was filled with glossy magazines, titled *Coping* and *Fit Pregnancy*.

A younger man, perhaps in his thirties, walked with the aid of a crutch, pulling his leg through with a swinging motion from the hip. His knee appeared locked straight. As he dropped onto a chair next to the fish aquarium, a receptionist came along and offered him a jumbo muffin.

"You're looking...you look great in navy blue," she said. Then she asked him if he was working this week.

"No. I'll be *here* this week, for treatment," he said. His tone rang negative.

"So, we get to see your smiling face all week?" she asked.

"I won't be smiling," he said.

I didn't know what kind of treatment he was referring to, but my heart ached for him. Harriette seemed to take her treatment in stride. Since she hadn't arrived yet, I decided to check out the artwork in the hallway. Among the frames on the wall I found a written piece:

> The "Wind Beneath My Wings" is my mother's and my song, because she is the wind beneath my wings. Where she gets her courage and energy from, nobody knows, but she spreads it to people wherever she goes.
>
> Though our life has been filled with sickness and grief, she manages to keep our family on our feet. This can't be taken literally because I am confined to a wheelchair.
>
> She would spend sleepless nights at my bedside either reading to me or playing games because I wasn't able to breathe. We moved across the country to try to make a better life for me. I have had numerous life threatening surgeries. My mother was always there. She taught me not to feel sorry for myself and not to allow my deteriorating condition to control my life.
>
> My mom has been my mentor, my teacher, my nurse, my case manager, and my best friend—my reason for wanting to stay alive.
>
> Several years ago my mom got breast cancer, but she told me not to worry because everything would be okay. Now she is fighting to stay alive with the cancer metastasized to her bones. This experience has taught us that nobody is immortal—not even my mom. We have learned to take one day at a time and use it as though it were our last.
>
> Her influence and support allowed me to become an accomplished artist whereby I can express my feelings. I live in constant pain, knowing that my condition will only get worse, but Mom is able to make me laugh and enjoy life. People think I am courageous and ask me where I get my strength, and I tell them to look to the wind beneath my wings.

There was no name at the end, but I knew the author was Cyndi. It answered, in a way, why Harriette was still with us when so many others with advanced breast cancer were not.

When Harriette arrived, there was no time to mention to her what I'd found. I assumed she knew about it anyway. We headed directly to one of the treatment rooms, where I set my books and bags on the floor. Harriette, however, turned around and left the room as quickly as we'd entered, to go make a telephone call. "I'll be right back," she called. "Don't let them hook you up."

When she returned, Rose, an oncology nurse with beautiful long red hair, was following. Harriette was already relaying her family's problems to Rose as she plopped into the easy chair and unclasped her two top buttons to expose her port. She opened her mouth in a wide grimace as Rose pushed a needle into the port. "It hurts when she doesn't use that freeze stuff," Harriette told me.

She admitted she was upset and worrying about Jeff, who'd just had surgery to repair a tear in his pectoral muscle. "He's been close to death with pneumonia," she exclaimed. As an athlete and cyclist in top physical condition, he'd shocked and frightened her when he developed breathing complications twenty-four hours after his operation. "He's never been sick like this before, though he's better now."

She mentioned that Stanley was having tests to determine whether he'd been having TIAs—transient ischemic attacks—and his doctors were checking to see whether he had frontal lobe atrophy. "And Cyndi's been having a personality conflict with one of her personal nursing assistants, and now she's developed a gynecological problem, too," she added, concluding the rundown on all the family members.

Harriette had done her workout this morning at 5:30 because she had to take Cyndi to get her teeth pulled and then drive Stanley to his medical appointment. She had just visited Jeff in the hospital down the street before coming here for her own treatment. Listening to all she accomplished in a day made me dizzy.

We watched Rose disconnect the syringe she used to draw blood from Harriette's port. Rose connected a tube to a bag of saline that would flush out the port before the Aredia and the chemo ran through. "I can't have them rush my drugs, or I'll get sick," Harriette reminded me. "I have too much to do to get sick. The Jewish Family Services are sending us food today, and I'm going to cook it for Thanksgiving."

Harriette said she usually brought work to do during her two hours here, or she read or made appointments and wrote them in her Day-Timer. "Mostly, I'm on the phone," she said.

We were nearing the end of our visit, so I joked with her. "Maybe God put you here to try to trick you into slowing down."

Harriette laughed. "Yeah, but, I'm winning because I won't slow down."

I smiled, shaking my head. I thought she was a hero.

CHAPTER 19

Bone Marrow Transplant Unit

Before I had cancer my understanding of bone marrow transplants was that they were a last ditch effort to save a person's life. I knew they were used in treatment for leukemia and breast cancer and that sometimes people didn't survive them. They sounded awful and frightened me.

During the days when I had been waiting to consult with the oncologist, worried as to whether I would need chemo, I read case histories of other women and would wonder, *Am I like this woman or that one? Will I ever need a transplant?* Some women with aggressive advanced disease had chosen this treatment out of desperation, and many of them died in spite of their transplant. I felt sorry for those women. But many of the books I read were outdated; perhaps things had changed and transplants had become more successful. I never believed I was a candidate for the procedure; however, I wasn't totally sure. Dr. McAleese had said my cancer was aggressive and multifocal.

When my oncologist proclaimed I was low risk for a recurrence and didn't need chemotherapy, I stopped worrying about bone marrow transplants. I had no reason to think about them anymore. And when I learned, sometime later, that studies reported (in spring of 1999) high-dose chemotherapy to be no more effective than standard chemotherapy, I vowed never to undergo a transplant—no matter what.

It had been almost two years since I'd given thought to this subject when I bumped into a neighbor I hadn't seen in years. We were both exiting the grocery store. Immediately my mind flashed back to the time in 1996 when I'd been shocked to see her name, Sue Niksic, listed in black marker on the wallboard in the University of Colorado Bone Marrow Transplant Unit. I had been working there on an interpreting assignment. On that hot summer day I had shivered, thinking that my young neighbor might have breast cancer. I'd thought only older women got it.

Although I didn't know at the time that there was a difference between stem cell transplants and bone marrow transplants, I knew they could be life threatening. I believed they had come about in the '80s and were still experimental as far as a last resort treatment for advanced breast cancer. They could cost up to $100,000, and many insurance companies refused to pay for them since they hadn't been established as an effective treatment for breast cancer. I shuddered to think that Sue had to go through this. She had small children.

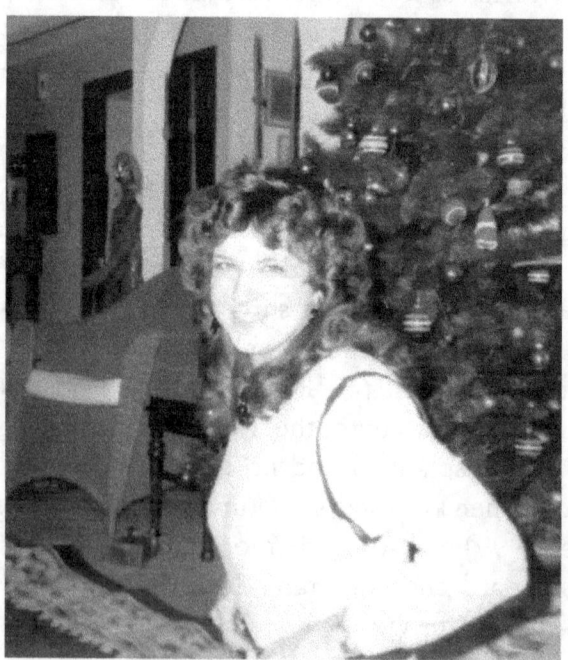

Sue Niksic, Christmas 1993

As we pushed our carts toward the parking lot, I thought to ask her, as if we both had cards to the same club, "Did you have a bone marrow transplant?"

"Yes," she said. "I had breast cancer when I was pregnant." Sue stopped her cart behind her car. Her son and daughter had been taking turns climbing in and out of her grocery basket as she pushed it. They seemed oblivious to our conversation. I told Sue I'd had breast cancer, too.

She seemed surprised. "My cancer's back now," she told me quietly. "It's in my liver. My kids don't know about it, and I don't want them to."

Obviously, the parking lot wasn't the best place for our conversation, so I asked Sue whether she would mind if I called her sometime. She said no, she didn't mind. So I promised I would.

I was eager to meet and talk with her again, but even though we lived an equivalent of only two city blocks from each other, it was difficult for us to arrange the time. Sue was busy fighting for her life. At the same time, she wasn't dwelling on only that. She had other priorities, such as her family and her community. With her time so focused, I didn't know whether we would ever be able to connect. Nevertheless, I hoped we would.

CHAPTER 20

To Lasso a Wild Horse

Harriette was busy fighting for her life, too. While her health and family issues occupied her, she had another objective—getting her story told, and it wasn't finished. Since it was through me that she was telling it, she began taking the initiative to get us together.

She planned me into her schedule and didn't let long periods of time go by in between our visits. Consequently, I spent more time with her than my other survivor friends. We met often, and I loved it. I was fascinated by Harriette and her cancer because she seemed to have defied all the odds. I wanted to understand how it was that *she* had survived nine years of metastatic cancer when many people survive only two years after a recurrence.

Recurrences, I was learning, were more challenging to treat than cancer confined to the breast tissue only because after cancer recurs there is no cure and recurrences can be sneaky. Sometimes, we don't recognize the symptoms because we don't want to, or we're too busy or too stressed. It may even be stress itself that brings on the recurrence. Doctors don't know. And they don't always recognize the symptoms of a recurrence either.

I saw all of these in Harriett's case when I asked her one day to tell me how hers came about. And I saw her dogged determination.

"When my cancer came back in 1992, I hadn't been thinking about it for several years," she said. "I'd been busy immersed in the business program at the community college in Aurora, raising Jeff, and taking care of Cyndi, who had been getting worse since 1987. Then, Stanley suffered a small stroke in 1989, which complicated things at home even more because all of a sudden he had difficulty learning new things and completing tasks. I had to start making lists to help keep him focused because he could get lost in a department store. But, I kept up with everything I had to do. I was so organized at the office that my supervisor bragged about me. At an awards dinner in 1990 she said, 'Harriette can do ten things at once and never drop the ball.' I took pride in my ability to do multiple tasks.

"Things started to change in February 1992, one month before my fiftieth birthday. I had begun training for a triathlon sponsored by the athletic center where I worked out. I was swimming laps every day, running, and biking around the neighborhood. It was going well at first, but after a couple of weeks, I started getting unusually fatigued and short of breath. The shortness of breath appeared every time I tried to exercise.

"It wasn't until a friend at the gym said something to me about my trouble breathing that I realized something must be wrong," Harriette said. "So I went to see Cyndi's pulmonary specialist. He treated me with steroids for activity-induced asthma, but the steroids didn't help. I still had trouble breathing.

"Then an annoying pain in my scapula appeared that wouldn't stop. I complained to my mother about it and another pain in my hip, and she said, 'You're just too old to be doing a triathlon.'

"Cyndi's hunch was that my cancer was back, so I had an X-ray. It didn't show anything unusual, so I thought maybe my mother was right. Maybe I was too old to do a triathlon, but I didn't stop training for it. I just ignored the pain."

When the fatigue and the pain in her scapula started to become unbearable, Harriette returned to her internist, who ran some blood tests, including a sedimentation rate, which detects inflammation in the body. "The tests revealed a slightly elevated sed rate, which should have been a red flag that something serious was going on," Harriette said, "but he just told me to get more rest. He referred me to a physical therapist, and I started going to her for range-of-motion exercises and heat and ice treatments.

"The physical therapy didn't help. Even though I was feeling awful, Cyndi and Jeff and I decided to go to Las Vegas to celebrate Cyndi's twenty-seventh birthday, which was coming up in March. We went during the end of February so it wouldn't interfere with the busy time of Jeff's aeration and fertilization business. We stayed four days at the beautiful Mirage Hotel and saw a few shows. They had an incredibly enticing pool, but my physical therapist had told me not to use my shoulder, so I couldn't swim. I didn't even get in. Jeff was the only one who swam because Cyndi was too sick, and she hated the heat in Las Vegas anyway.

"Cyndi could still walk a little bit at that time, but she was using a wheelchair more and more. Jeff and I were taking turns lifting her, but mostly it was me, helping her with pivot transfers from the chair to the car and in the bedroom and bathroom. I was lifting her about ten times a day.

"I was exhausted when we got back to Denver, so I returned to the doctor. He told me I had the flu, and when I went back to work, still fatigued, people kept telling me I was saying *ouch* all the time. I kept on going, anyway, pushing through the pain and the fatigue.

"Then, in April, the Hartwood Athletic Center Master's Swim Team began training for a three-day meet to be held in Boulder. I wanted to compete with them, so I started training with them. In the pool I was struggling with my breathing, but I wouldn't give up. I kept going to the training for a couple of weeks. In May, on the weekend of the meet, I met up with the team in Boulder, and we trained on Friday night and a good part of Saturday in final preparation for the race on Sunday.

"At the end of the training we were practicing our dives when suddenly I heard a loud crack in my head and felt a snap in my neck. In the morning I woke up with pain so bad I was unable compete in the race. I even had trouble driving home that afternoon because I couldn't turn my head. I figured I'd just injured my neck somehow in the dive. We had a neck brace at home, left over from something, so I put it on and wore it to work the next day."

The hospital where Harriette worked specialized in spinal cord injuries, so she was able to joke with her coworkers when she walked into the office that morning wearing the brace. "I said, 'Look guys, I could have been a patient here.' I didn't know yet that I had actually sustained a pathologic fracture of my cervical vertebra. I just continued to wear the brace."

She'd been wearing it for a couple of days when her brother called from New York to tell her their father was in the Long Island Jewish Hospital emergency room. He'd suffered a brain aneurysm. "When I hung up the phone, I immediately started making arrangements to go there. I needed someone to help with Cyndi while I was gone."

At the hospital in New York, her father lay motionless, hooked up to an IV. "My brother and I agreed to take him off the life support, but they wouldn't do it for several days, until his doctor returned from vacation. I told my brother, 'I can only stay here for a week because Cyndi's too sick and I have to get back to work.' I spent the next few days there fighting with New York lawyers over the validity of the power of attorney for my father. I had the papers drawn up here in Colorado, and they argued that my power of attorney wasn't valid in New York.

"My father passed away two days after the doctor took him off the life support, and we held the funeral the next day. I came home Sunday, worn out and in terrible pain. I thought it was from all the fighting with the lawyers.

"In the shower that night I suddenly knew what was wrong when I discovered a new lump on my chest. When Stanley came into the bedroom while I was dressing, I told him, 'I know why I'm so tired and in so much pain. The cancer is back.'

"Both of us were worried, and so I called my surgeon on Monday morning. When he saw me, he said, 'It's superficial—probably just a benign cyst. We'll take it out. Don't worry.' His receptionist scheduled me for a minor procedure the following Monday."

Four days later Harriette had more alarming symptoms. "I had severe pain bothering me while I was at work. It was Friday—the day of our spring field day at the hospital."

While all the staff and spinal cord patients were on their way outside to enjoy some food and fun, Judy told Harriette to call her oncologist. "I tried to contact Dr. Garfield, but I could only leave a message with his nurse." While they waited, Judy and Harriette joined the others outside.

They sat eating baked beans and potato salad, squinting in the sun while patients in wheelchairs threw balls at the dunk tank target. Every time one of them hit the target, the crowd broke out in wild cheers, as their victims, the doctors, got dumped from their seats into the icy water. Even fraught with worry, Harriette and Judy laughed when the doctors emerged from the tank, sopping wet.

"Finally, Dr. Garfield called and said he was leaving for Europe soon to go on vacation, so I should come in right away. I sped to his office, and he found another lump—in my armpit. And on the X-ray he saw spots on my lungs and spine. 'It doesn't look good,' he said. 'We'll need to schedule you for a minor procedure and get a bone scan in the next week.' He asked if I wanted him to call my husband or someone else.

"I said, 'Yes, call Judy.' When he got her on the telephone, he told her what we already suspected. My cancer was back, in explosive metastasis. Then he handed me the phone. I asked Judy, 'How am I going to tell my kids?'

"Judy always had ideas. She said, 'Maybe we could all go to the temple tonight and have the Rabbi help you tell them.' The Rabbi at Temple Sinai was great at that kind of stuff. So Judy called him and asked if we could all meet there."

Harriette's family didn't normally go to temple during the week, so something seemed odd to Cyndi and Jeff when Harriette insisted they go there that evening. She told them there was something she needed to talk to them about.

"After the services were over, we gathered in a corner of the social hall with the Rabbi. He told our kids my cancer was back.

He said something like this was just a few bumps in the road, trying to give them encouragement and hope. Cyndi started screaming immediately, and Jeff began crying hysterically. I didn't cry, though, and Stanley didn't cry either because he already knew."

As Harriette continued her story, she impressed me with how she fulfilled obligations no matter what the obstacles were. Although I hadn't experienced a recurrence, I saw bits of myself in her swirl of anger, denial, and acceptance and how she tried to maintain control when she was feeling out of control.

The day after she got the traumatic news of her recurrence, she showed up to fulfill her volunteer assignment for the Max Fund, the animal protection society, where she was to help man their booth at the Capital Hill People's Fair. This is Denver's annual arts and crafts festival celebrating urban diversity. Exhibitors in tents line the lawns in front of Civic Center Park, displaying unique handmade crafts and dispensing information on various issues.

While the sun beat down, intensifying aromas of cinnamon roasted almonds, barbequed turkey legs, and old country kettle corn, Harriette stood under the sign that read, "No Kill Animal Shelter." Crowds of people passed by and walked up and down the aisles between the booths. Some people stopped to pick up brochures from her table. Others lingered to chat about the organization dedicated to injured animals.

"In the heat, the chain around my neck was clinging to my skin," Harriette said. "When I reached up to wipe the perspiration and rearrange the chain, I found another lump."

At the nape was another nodule on her spine. "Now I had three, and my surgeon was only expecting to remove one, but I had to wait until Monday until I could call him.

"He was surprised to hear from me when I called, and he said, 'I don't think we have enough time tomorrow to remove all three.'"

He wanted to reschedule, but Harriette was adamant. "I said no, I want all three of them removed tomorrow, and I want a local anesthetic because I want to go back to work." So the surgeon removed all three of the nodules on the same day at Swedish Hospital. Afterward, Harriette, Judy, and Stanley waited for the results. The news came a few hours later: malignant—all three of them. They were identified as adenocarcinoma, a cancer that originates in glandular tissues such as the breasts.

"We'd already known it was bad," Harriette said, "but I was stunned. I said, 'Wow. This could kill me.'"

Waves of disbelief came in between reassurances to herself. "I kept saying, I'm going to be okay. I can do this. Later on, other people kept telling me I was going to be okay, but it bothered me when they said that. I wanted to say to them, *how the hell do you know? I* wanted to be the one to tell *them* I was going to be okay."

After the confirmation of her malignancy came, a bone scan was scheduled to determine the extent of metastasis. If there were more cancerous tumors on her bones, the scan would show the areas as "hot spots." If there were metastases in her liver and lungs, they wouldn't show on a bone scan. Blood tests and chest X-rays could be used to identify those as well as CT scans and MRIs, which were also useful in identifying metastasis to the brain. CT scans and MRIs were expensive, however, and would expose her to more radiation. They weren't necessary at the moment.

Later that week Harriette returned to the hospital, to the nuclear medicine department, where a technician injected a radioactive substance into her bloodstream. "I had to drink a lot of water for the next two hours while they waited for the isotope to circulate throughout my body. Then they put me under a machine that took a picture of my skeleton."

The radioactive liquid concentrated in areas of the bone where there was increased metabolism like there was with arthritis or a fracture or cancer. The machine read the number of radioactive particles, and areas of concern showed up as white spots on the picture. The water aided the isotope's circulation as well as helped to wash it out of her system.

"A few days later, I sat in Dr. Garfield's office, staring at the picture of my bones, and I said, 'I don't know what I'm looking at.'

Dr. Garfield replied, 'You don't want any white spots.' The scan was mostly white, and I knew I was in deep trouble then. The picture looked like a lit-up Christmas tree."

There were tumors on her neck, hips, spine, pelvis, and skull—all the key places breast cancer likes to migrate. Doctors were almost powerless fighting recurrences like these, and people who suffered from them usually only survived six months to two years.

"Dr. Garfield admitted my prognosis was not at all good. He said, 'This is like trying to lasso a wild horse.'"

It was a grim picture—terminal. Yet her story was not over.

CHAPTER 21

Terminal

―――◆―――

With a prognosis of "terminal," things indeed look grim. Yet within us are natural instincts for survival and hope. Without hope, there is no fight to survive, and without a fight, there is no hope. I already knew Harriette was a fighter, but as her story unfolded, I saw this even more. In spite of her dismal prognosis she had much working in her favor. She was strong, emotionally and physically, and she had a competitive spirit. Also in her favor was an arsenal of new drugs and hormones that were beginning to make long-term control of breast cancer possible. There was hope.

So she began her fight, first with tamoxifen. With all of her tumors testing ER positive, Harriette stood a chance that it would block her body's natural estrogen, the fuel source, from her tumors. The oncologist started her on the hormone right away, in hopes of shrinking her tumors, along with mega-doses of Decadron. If there was a tumor pressing on her spinal cord, it could cause paralysis. The high dose steroids would reduce the swelling near the bone fractures and prevent this.

Hospitalized and hooked up to an IV, Harriette's hope wavered. "I thought I might not have long to live," she said, "so I asked the nurses for a typewriter. I wanted to compile some information and instructions for my family—things that they would need to know when I was gone.

"I started typing but didn't finish it. Later that night, I was so wired and unable to sleep from the Decadron, I put my robe over my hospital gown and pushed my IV pole through the tunnel between Swedish Hospital and Craig Hospital to my office. I had many things to do. I was a workaholic, and I was used to working at night anyway, so I wanted to be there. My office was my sanctuary, the place where I always felt comfort and solace."

Harriette worked at her desk for over an hour and then pushed her IV pole through the tunnel again, back to her hospital room where she finished eight pages of typed instructions to her family. On Monday she was discharged from the hospital and went back to work.

"At home I still found it hard to sleep, due to the steroids. One night I sat alone reviewing the list of important things I wanted my family to know and the strict budget I'd drawn up for them. Suddenly, out of fear, anger, and frustration, I tore all the papers into tiny pieces and threw them up into the air. They fell like ticker tape. I'd decided I was not giving in to this enemy. I was going to keep the promise I made to my family years ago, that I would always be around for them—because they needed me."

Harriette continued taking the tamoxifen for one month. But things got worse. "Stanley and I were planning to go to New York for Stan's cousin's Bat Mitzvah in July. We'd been looking forward to the extravagant party. We were all packed and ready to leave for the airport in the morning, and then I woke up with intense pain. Stanley said, 'Are you sure we can go?' I said, 'I'm not sure.'"

They decided she had better call the oncologist. It was seven o'clock on Saturday morning, but they thought there should be a doctor on call. "I told Stanley, 'If it's my doctor who calls back, I'll go in, but if it's not, we're going to the airport.'

"It was my doctor who was on call. He told me I needed to get in for an X-ray. I said, 'But we're going to New York. I have to catch a plane!'"

Dr. Garfield countered with, "It's best if you can get over there right away." He told Harriette to put her luggage in the car. So, instead of going to the airport, Stanley drove her to the hospital for the X-ray.

The picture revealed pathologic and compression fractures on the second cervical and ninth thoracic vertebrae. The spontaneous bone fractures were typical of bone metastases. The shortness of breath she had was typical of metastases to the lungs.

"Dr. Garfield said I had to be admitted to the hospital right away. I needed an oophorectomy (removal of the ovaries) to reduce the estrogen in my body. We never made it to the airport. I was mad because we weren't able to go to New York, and I was upset we had to miss the Bat Mitzvah. I was angry that if the estrogen was the cause of my cancer, then why hadn't an oophorectomy been done seven years ago?"

The procedure was done by laparoscopy on the following Friday. "I was supposed to go home afterward, but they couldn't stabilize my blood pressure, so they had to admit me overnight."

An orderly wheeled Harriette from the operating room on a gurney out to the elevator. From the elevator he wheeled her onto the oncology floor. "When we rolled onto the new wing of Rose Hospital, I glimpsed the sign that said "Terminal," and I thought, *I don't belong on this side.*"

The doctor said Harriette would need radiation and chemotherapy and that he would think over the weekend about which drug regimen would be the most effective. She went home the next morning and was back to work on Monday.

Before she began going for her chemotherapy at the old Cancer Center, Hematology Oncology Associates on Franklin Street, where they had huge fish tanks and only curtains for privacy, Harriette admitted she felt scared. "I was searching for options. I wasn't sure I wanted that strange stuff going into my body, and I didn't know what to do.

"I'd heard that Dr. Jones was doing Bone Marrow Transplants (BMT) at University Hospital at that time, so Judy and I went to consult with a second oncologist, for another opinion, to see if I might be a candidate for a BMT. His opinion was that I was making a very big mistake if I chose the radiation and chemotherapy. Very abruptly he said, 'You won't make it six months if you don't get the transplant.'"

After the consultation Judy and Harriette went back to their office and called the Dana-Farber Cancer Center in Boston to seek advice. "The opinion of the experts at Dana-Farber was that I might be too old for the BMT. I was fifty years old, and their criteria had an age cutoff at fifty. But since I was an athlete and had been in good shape, they thought it might be possible for me."

When Harriette talked to them again, however, they had changed their minds. Their opinion now was that she was not a good candidate because her cancer was too advanced. They thought she wouldn't survive the transplant because she was so weak and could hardly walk because of the pain in her spine. "They didn't think I would live too long. So I started the chemotherapy and radiation. I had to psych myself up for the chemotherapy by saying it was my energy juice."

Her oncologist had decided to start her on a regimen of 5FU along with Leucovorin, the binding agent that makes the 5FU work better. The drugs would be administered through a vein, every week. She would taper off from the steroids. "It was late July, and Dr. Garfield had said if the chemotherapy worked, it would probably stop working after a while and that I probably had between four months to two years to live. I would be on chemotherapy for the remainder of my life."

CHAPTER 22

The Miracle Drug

One month after starting chemotherapy, Harriette began radiation treatments. It had been almost eight years since her first radiation, and now they were hoping to shrink the painful tumors on her spine, hip, and neck. As she started down this path, Harriette prayed it would work because she believed this was all there was for her. Neither Harriette nor her doctor knew about Aredia yet.

Harriette described to me what that point in time was like. "Radiation was difficult. My first radiation treatments had been easy compared to this time. I had to hold still in several different, awkward positions on the table. I remember lying there in pain, thinking of the movie *Love Story*, where Ali MacGraw's character dies from leukemia. The scene where she was at a baseball game played vividly in my mind. She was wrapped up in a blanket, bald and freezing, sitting on the bleachers. I remembered watching that movie in 1970, thinking, I hope that doesn't happen to me someday."

After the radiation beams ceased, Harriette couldn't get up from the table because of the excruciating pain in her neck. "Even with four people helping me, I nearly passed out. It took several minutes until I could catch my breath."

For six weeks she endured the daily radiation and the painfully awkward positions. By October her hair had thinned to half its normal thickness. She was sick and weak from the chemotherapy, radiation, and trying to work but refused to give in to being ill. She spoke of the other radiation patients in the waiting room of Porter Hospital as if she weren't one of them. "I said, 'I don't look sick like they do.'"

In actuality, Harriette looked worse. She was now losing nearly two pounds a day and had gone from 142 pounds down to 112. "I couldn't eat because food tasted like cardboard," Harriette said. "All I could tolerate was Jell-O, oatmeal, and soup."

She was so weak she had trouble getting out of the car. At work she had no energy to climb the stairs from the cafeteria to her first-floor office. Instead of giving in to the fatigue and using the elevator to get back to her office, she pulled herself up the stairs by the banister, one step at a time.

Concerned, her doctor recommended they insert an Infusaport under her skin to make the weekly treatments easier to administer. Harriette had the surgeon do the procedure as an outpatient in a morning, with a local anesthetic, so she wouldn't miss work in the afternoon. For two grueling hours the surgeon wrestled with the port's insertion. With it finally placed, snuggly, above where her right breast had been, Harriette did go to work that afternoon. The port would eventually last an unheard of seven years before it failed.

By December, instead of feeling better, Harriette was feeling worse. Nevertheless, she forced herself to go into work every day until one morning she caved from her dogged determination not to be sick. "I finally admitted to myself that I felt horrible. I called the doctor from work, and he told me to come in to see him. But he couldn't find anything wrong with me, so I thought I must just be imagining things."

On the drive back to her office, every inhalation caused a stabbing pain. But the doctor had found nothing wrong. She worried that if she complained to the people at work, they would think she was a hypochondriac. At her desk she sat staring blankly at stacks of papers, wondering whether her pains were real, when someone interrupted her thoughts. "It was my boss," Harriette said. "She said, 'Your color looks awful.'

"That evening, in spite of feeling terrible, I dragged myself to my cancer support group. I never liked to miss a meeting. The nurses in the group told me that I didn't look good, and then one of them left immediately to go call my doctor. He was still in his office at 6:30, and he said for me to come in right away."

An X-ray showed two large pulmonary emboli, either one of which could kill her at any minute. "The doctor said I must to go to Presbyterian St. Luke's hospital right away, but I told him if I had to go into a hospital, I was going to Swedish Hospital." He didn't argue. He just said, 'Then don't make any stops on the way. Just get there.' So I drove myself to Swedish and was admitted for treatment."

The emboli, they said, were caused by the port surgery she'd had two months previously. People with active cancer are prone to pulmonary emboli, she was told. Harriette was put on mega-doses of heparin to dissolve the blood clots and then therapeutic doses of Coumadin to keep her blood thin.

"They told me I would be on Coumadin for the rest of my life, as well, and I would have to have the levels checked frequently for fluctuations. My blood can't be too thick because it might create new clots, and it can't be too thin or it will cause hemorrhages.

"I stayed in the hospital that time for eight days, and I dressed in my clothes every day. The nurses said to me, 'It's like you're not even sick.'" It was denial mixed with determinism.

As she was recovering from the life-threatening embolism, Harriette's family thought she would benefit from a short leisure trip, so, at the end of December, she and Jeff took a four-day cruise from Miami Beach. "I was nauseated and sick the whole time," she said, "but I made the best of it, and we danced on the ship until two in the morning.

"When we returned after the cruise, a doctor from work showed me an article about some clinical trials with an osteoporosis medication that was being tested to see if it reduced pain and fractures in breast cancer that had spread to the bones."

The article described a drug that halts hypercalcemia, a condition that often occurs with cancer, where calcium seeps from the bones, causing them to weaken. Too much calcium in the blood also causes nausea, thirst, irregular heartbeat, confusion, and, in severe cases, kidney failure and coma. The drug slows the breakdown of bone where the cancer is trying to grow, giving it less space, thus inhibiting the tumor's growth. As well as reducing the chance for bone fractures, the drug reduces the pain in the bones.

"I showed the article to Dr. Garfield and told him I wasn't interested in the trial," Harriette explained. "I just wanted the medication."

The medication was called Aredia. Although Harriette and Dr. Garfield both were aware the drug didn't necessarily work for everyone, he agreed she should try it. She would get the drug once a month by infusion for six months, just as indicated for the clinical trial.

Shortly after she began her course with Aredia, Harriette started seeing articles in the newspaper about Ocean Journey, a giant aquarium being built in Denver, which was to open in 1999. "At first, I felt remorse that I might never get to visit the aquarium," Harriette said. "But then I began to visualize myself on opening day, going to see the exotic aquatic life. We had received a fundraising solicitation in the mail, to buy a drop of the ocean to help build the aquarium, so my family purchased one. We got a card that said, 'U made it, Ca survivor,' and it had my name on it. I became an Ocean Journey Charter Member, which meant when the aquarium opened, I would have free admission for a year."

As one month on Aredia grew into two and then into four, when Harriette was alone, she would often scream out, "I want to live!" When six months passed, Harriette was not dead from her cancer. She was alive. As time went by she began to awaken to the fact that she was not dying. She found herself trying to understand what had happened to her and why. "I thought cancer was supposed to change people," she said, "but it hadn't changed me. I had been living my life exactly as I'd always done. I had been driven to keep working and to keep everything in my life going the same. Then I thought, maybe this recurrence was a two-by-four hitting me over the head so I would stop and think—live my life differently.

"I started to reevaluate my life. But I didn't want to do anything differently. I had Cyndi to take care of, and I still wanted to work. I loved to work. So, I decided not to take away anything in my life, but to *add* something. We would travel."

The Grobers had been accustomed to living on a tight budget, with money specifically allocated for food and rent, telephone and cleaning, haircuts and entertainment, and most importantly, emergencies. They'd always saved for *years* for vacations. Now, they would forget about the budget and start taking trips. "I realized that it was okay for us, for *me* especially, to take a vacation without Cyndi," Harriette said. "Stanley and I had been planning a trip for our thirtieth anniversary in November. But in September, the doctor said, 'Don't wait,' so we went two months early."

An aide came in to help with Cyndi's care. Then, while Harriette's mother came and stayed at the house, the anniversary couple flew to California and took a Greyhound Bus Tour from Los Angeles to San Francisco.

"I was already weak and feeling sick while we were at San Simone for the tour of the Hearst Castle, and later on I was feeling even worse at Monterey Bay, so Stanley thought we should skip the last tour—of Alcatraz—because of all the stairs. But I was determined to see it, so we did." They finished the trip, including Alcatraz, and flew home.

Six months later Harriette was still alive and getting stronger. It appeared that the Aredia was the miracle drug, so she started living again—with zest.

"Though my tumors had not totally disappeared, they had stopped growing, and I had less pain, so we took another trip to Florida in March of '94. Jeff went with us on that trip. He was twenty-six then. We visited Epcot, Disney World, and MGM. Then we started taking two trips a year for the next four years.

"The trips were difficult in the beginning because I felt I needed to do the things that were important to me while I still could, yet I grappled with the guilt of leaving Cyndi behind. We went anyway, and we visited Cancun, twice. Jeff and I swam with the dolphins at an amusement park there. It was not exactly like what we had imagined doing at Key West; still, we got to hold onto the dolphins' fins in a big tank while they soared through the water at seventy miles per hour. It was exhilarating. And then the dolphin master snapped his fingers in the air, and the dolphin stopped on a dime—just short of hitting the wall of the tank."

In Cancún they visited the Mayan ruins at Chichen Itza, where Harriette and Jeff climbed the steps of the El Castillo pyramid. The ninety-one steps were so narrow they practically had to crawl to get to the top of the thousand-year-old structure. "Jeff was afraid we would fall or that someone else in the crowd of people on the steps would fall and come tumbling down on top of us.

"After that trip Stanley and I blew money like crazy for four more years. We went on more trips, to Alaska and Hawaii. We went to Mexico again and snorkeled at Cozumel and Key West. We didn't save any money for emergencies like we used to."

Another life change Harriette made during that time was adding biking to her regular regimen of swimming and weightlifting. She and Jeff joined the Denver Bicycle Touring Club, a group that rode together four times a week. Jeff and Harriette started riding with the group on weekends and every Tuesday night. With a leader, the group rides through mountain towns for thirty miles or so, and then they stop to eat in Chinese or Mexican restaurants. Along with that, Harriette and Jeff began their own biking tradition. Every year in the first week of August they biked the canyon in Glenwood Springs, swam in the world's largest hot springs pool, and stayed overnight at a hotel. Sometimes they stayed at the Hot Springs Lodge. What began as one overnight in time turned into a four-night bike trip, including time set for hiking, swimming, shopping, and a favorite stop of theirs—the Aspen Music Festival, where they dropped in on a piano concerto or a recital by one of the world's finest musicians.

"On the ride back from Frisco to Breckenridge, it's always raining," Harriette said. "Because we enjoy ourselves, we wait too long to head back and always get caught in the afternoon rain.

"These were positive changes for me, but they did come at a price. Before my recurrence, I had always included Cyndi in our activities. Now I was engaged in interests of my own, and Cyndi's and my close relationship began to deteriorate till it finally became intolerable. We were fighting all the time. It took a long time and a lot of counseling to bring us back together."

In the meantime IV chemotherapy had become a way of life for Harriette, along with its side effects. Although she never lost her hair completely, she no longer had eyebrows or eyelashes, her skin was dry, her fingernails were lined and cracked, and her toenails had come off completely. Her eyes were dry and frequently became infected and crusty from clogged tear ducts. Every morning she had to steam and soften them with hot washcloths. She was annoyed by a racing heart rate and migraine headaches from lack of sleep. And there was constant fatigue. Later, after three years on chemotherapy, short-term memory problems began to crop up.

In spite of the problems associated with the side effects, Harriette carried on an active life, fitting in volunteer work around her treatments. She visited women newly diagnosed with breast cancer as a Reach to Recovery volunteer, something she had begun doing in 1986 after her own mastectomies. "I felt I was given a second chance at life for a reason, and I needed to give something back to my community," Harriette said. "I wanted to make a difference in other people's lives, so I started volunteering at the zoo and for the Max Fund animal shelter." She would also begin to tutor first-grade students in reading at an elementary School and become an usher with Stanley at the Denver Center Theater.

By this time, after spending so many hours with Harriette, I was beginning to realize how much I was learning from her, not only about her and her cancer, but also about myself, about human nature, and about how precious life is. When we have a brush with death, we take a second look at how we are living. From that new perspective, we don't put off for tomorrow what we can do today.

We start doing all of our living now. And we look for ways to make a difference somehow, so that our lives mean something.

After we come out from a personal crisis, in control after the chaos, we have energy to focus outside of ourselves again. We want to effect positive change so others may benefit from our experience. We get involved. We do things we never did before. Harriette got involved in the politics of breast cancer.

As I'd been reading and learning about the history of breast cancer, Harriette opened my eyes to the politics. She told me about the Colorado Breast Cancer Coalition, which she joined in 1993, a year after her recurrence, and she introduced me to Anne Weiher, a friend who was the coordinator of the coalition at that time.

From Anne Weiher I found out more about the grassroots advocacy group and Harriette's role in it when she and I met for lunch one day. Anne explained to me that the coalition was aligned with the National Breast Cancer Coalition (NBCC), which was established in 1991 to educate and teach patients how to become effective advocates. "When Harriette joined the coalition," Anne said, "we were working to galvanize people around Colorado in support of state legislation that would require insurance companies to cover cancer patients who were participating in clinical trials. Harriette started to help us in trying to get the bill passed. Then, in the spring of '94, she volunteered to be the secretary for the group.

"At that time, Harriette didn't look too good, and people were concerned," Anne said. "Another member of the coalition called me and said, 'I don't think Harriette should be the secretary; I don't think she's gonna make it through the summer.' Everyone thought Harriette was dying, and they thought she was in denial because she was making plans for the future. But I didn't think that was a good enough reason to not let her take the secretary job, so we gave it to her. For two more years she helped us as we tried to get the bill passed on reimbursement for cancer patients involved in clinical trials, but the bill failed, twice."

As Anne portrayed what was happening at that time, I was picturing Harriette at those meetings. In my mind I saw her, thin and gray of pallor, showing up to each coalition meeting with pen and paper in hand. The image quickly faded when Anne said, "As it turned out, Harriette was the first and only recording secretary, serving during the entire life of the coalition from 1994–2000. She took the minutes of the meetings and kept records. She worked on the development of the *Breast Cancer Resource Directory*, using funds someone had bequeathed to the coalition. She assisted in the newsletter production and later worked on the information hotline."

Harriette's employer at Craig Hospital looked favorably on her involvement with the coalition and allowed her time for its activities. That support, along with a scholarship from the National Breast Cancer Coalition, enabled Harriette to fly to New Orleans to participate in Project LEAD (Leadership, Education, and Advocacy Development) in 1996. With thirty other attendees over five exhausting days, she learned about science and epidemiology related to breast cancer. As a layperson she was trained on the clinical aspects of breast cancer and scientific research. She gained knowledge about policy development. From there she could expand her advocacy into the scientific and medical communities.

"I'm a Project LEAD graduate, too," Anne continued. "Graduates can sit on panels with doctors and scientists and have influence on decisions regarding the use of research funding." As LEAD graduates, Anne had served in this capacity by reviewing grant proposals, and Harriette had traveled to Washington, D.C., in 1997, 1998, and 1999, on scholarships and grants, to join members of the NBCC in their annual Advocacy Training Conference. With hundreds of advocates from across the country, Harriette attended sessions on becoming an informed and effective lobbyist. The participants were briefed on the coalition's legislative priorities and taught how bills were passed. The workshops prepared them for Lobby Day on Capitol Hill, the last day of the conference, where they met with legislators in an effort to effect change on public policies related to breast cancer.

The next time I met with Harriette, she seemed pleased when I told her what I'd learned from Anne about Project LEAD. "I was never political before I went to Project LEAD," Harriette said. "But it became part of my bargaining with my greater power. The two greatest fears I'd always had were public speaking and death. It wasn't that I was afraid to die; it was just that I didn't want to. So, I bargained that if I were allowed to live, I would do something to make this a better place. Even though I'm not too comfortable speaking to groups, I learned to be persuasive to legislators."

So that she could help all women in this fight, Harriette became an advocate. With fellow Colorado breast cancer survivors, Lois Hjelmstad and Vicki Tosher, she met with legislators on Capitol Hill. Harriette scheduled all the meetings for the Colorado delegates to speak with the senators and representatives about NBCC's legislative priorities. They had discussions with Senator Ben Nighthorse Campbell and Representatives Diana DeGette and Joel Hefley. They met with other representatives' healthcare aides. "Vicki did most of the talking in those meetings," Harriette said. "She was the most dynamic force among us and the most influential to the legislators when she told them, 'Between the three of us, we have only one breast.'"

Their efforts did effect some positive changes. "We got them to move on the CDC bill (Centers for Disease Control)," Harriette stated proudly. "They had already passed the Breast and Cervical Cancer Mortality Prevention Act in 1990, the law that allows free screening for detection of cervical and breast cancer for indigent women. But then these women had no money to pay for their treatment after they were diagnosed. We went back to Washington in 1998 and again in 1999 to push for legislation to provide federal aid for their treatment—through Medicaid."

The efforts of the National Breast Cancer Coalition would eventually lead to President Clinton's signing into law the Breast and Cervical Cancer Prevention and Treatment Act of 2000. By then, however, Harriette's involvement with the coalition had diminished. Her life had become too complicated by Cyndi's illness. Instead of traveling to Washington each spring, Harriette kept her advocacy work on a local level. She began serving on the Breast Cancer Task Force and the Public Issues Committee of the American Cancer Society in Denver.

In the spring of 1996 Harriette's advocacy fanned outward in style after she heard about the upcoming Danskin Women's Triathlon Series. A staff person at the Rocky Mountain Cancer Center mentioned it to her. "You have to do this," the woman said to her. The triathlon was to be held at Cherry Creek State Park in the month of August. It was for women of all shapes and sizes and of varying degrees of abilities, from ages fourteen through seventy. A percentage of all the entry fees was going to the Susan G. Komen Breast Cancer Foundation, an organization dedicated to finding the cure for breast cancer. The woman told Harriette that the registration was free for survivors entering for the first time.

With her athletic spirit, Harriette was always game for a challenge, and this was for a worthy cause, so she began training in earnest for the Triathlon. The actual event would require her to swim half a mile in the murky Cherry Creek Reservoir, bike twelve miles, part of it across the dam, and run a five-kilometer trail. By August, however, the effects of continuous doses of chemotherapy were becoming evident. Harriette was run down and sick. "I was actually toxic from the drugs, and I knew it, but I showed up for the triathlon anyway," she told me.

Thousands of people were there. The athletes began with the swim and were permitted into the water in waves of 75–150 women, starting with the twenty-year-olds or the "most fit." "There was hardly any place to park your bike while we did the swim," Harriette remembered. "I was in the 'fifty-and-up' age group, and our bikes were in the last row. We were the last group to enter the water, and since I'm a pool swimmer, with ropes and lanes, the open water was very scary for me."

At first, the water was icy cold and took her breath away. She warmed as she swam although she had to bring her head up often to look out over the water to keep on course. Swimming alongside so many people, she found if she took a breath at the wrong time, she got a splash of water in her lungs.

"The swim was tough," Harriette said. "About one-third of the way, my pulse rate was going way faster than normal because of the chemotherapy, and I was thinking about grabbing onto one of the buoys and quitting. I did hold on to one of them to rest for a bit, but I didn't quit." She finished the swim and, although she felt totally drained, she made her way to her bike. "The biking was the easiest part for me. I was used to biking at the reservoir. The hardest part was the run because I don't normally run. My legs felt like rubber, so I walked most of it. Then I started running during the last quarter mile so people would think I ran the whole thing."

Toward the end of the run Harriette fought against nausea and intense exhaustion. Still, she pushed on, saying to herself, *"You can do it, you can do it."* Crossing the finish line, she looked so drawn and pale that her own husband didn't even recognize her. "I ended up placing third in my age group. Afterward, a newspaper reporter interviewed me—I guess because I looked so old or so terrible, and later that evening I was on TV. I didn't remember any of it." For her efforts Harriette won a Danskin top and a pair of shorts. The reward for Harriette was not in the prize. The reward was that she'd done it.

Subsequently, because of her poor condition, Dr. Garfield lowered her drug dose. "The change in medication was scary," Harriette said, "but he figured out I was becoming toxic." It became a process of trial and error that would stretch on into years. What Dr. Garfield had said would *probably* be six months of IV chemotherapy surprised everyone as the years turned and kept on turning.

Enduring long-term chemotherapy, Harriette continued to challenge herself. She believed if she could lift five more pounds or swim a little faster, then she was definitely okay. Many times she discovered she had pushed herself too far. She had pressed on until she was overcome with dehydration and exhaustion.

"I would be so tired, I couldn't even talk. It started happening regularly." With fever and electrolytes all out of balance, she would wind up in the hospital, on IV fluids for a few days. "Eventually, I had to learn how to slow down and pay attention to my body. I've learned to do visualization exercises to help me relax and deal with managing my family and my life. Since then I haven't had to go into the hospital anymore.

"By 1997 we had spent all of our money on traveling," Harriette said, "and it seemed clear I was surviving cancer, so we had to stop all of the traveling and go back on a budget. I wanted to have some money to fall back on in an emergency, and we needed to buy a van to make it easier to transport Cyndi. Since I was getting better, I quit paying the premiums on the extra Life Insurance policies I'd taken out. It didn't look like we would need that additional coverage after all. I started setting that money aside for a trip later on. When the time for that trip eventually came, Cyndi was too sick, so we stayed home."

Harriette attributed her second chance on life to the Aredia, and two years after discontinuing the drug, she suffered another bone fracture, this time in her hip joint. It was in the ischium—one of the pelvic bones. Consequently, Dr. Garfield put her back on Aredia. By then, the National Cancer Institute had the results of the study on Aredia. The drug had shown it was completely able to stop tumor growth in some people, and so it had become standard protocol in treatment of bone metastases of breast cancer. Harriette would stay on the miracle drug indefinitely.

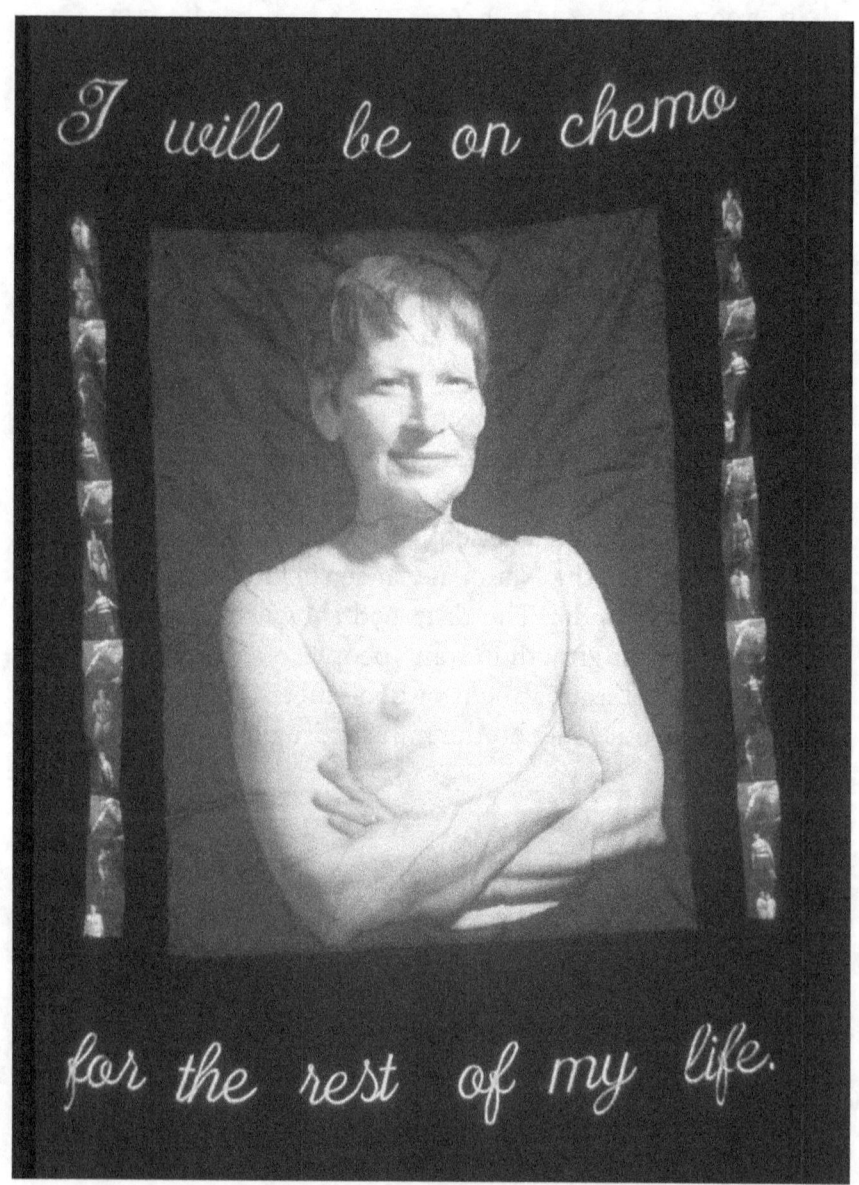

Harriette's *common threads* quilt

Photo by Cynthia O'Dell

CHAPTER 23

Common Threads

Over time, as Harriette recounted her story, I learned of another silent yet powerful role she had played in advocating the cause of breast cancer. She casually blurted out one day, "I'm on one of the quilts in *common threads*."

"What's that?" I asked.

"It's a nude picture of me that's on the road." Besides her profile in *MAMM* magazine, where she had become nationally recognized in 2001, Harriette had helped make a national social statement on breast cancer three years before, in 1998. She was one of the featured figures in this traveling quilt exhibit created by a University of Colorado graduate student.

I asked Harriette where I could see the exhibit, so I could understand better what she was talking about, but unfortunately it was no longer on display in Colorado. She put me in touch with the artist, Cynthia O'Dell, instead. I was disappointed that I would not get to see the quilts, except in pictures, but, between Cynthia, Harriette, and Anne Weiher, I put together the story of *common threads*.

From her home in Indiana, Cynthia shared with me over the telephone how *common threads* had been conceived and came to be. "I was in graduate school at the University of Colorado in Boulder, in 1996," Cynthia said, "working on a photography project about breast cancer for my master's thesis. I had already created a body of artwork centered on the theme of breasts and their significance in our culture, which I called my 'Breast Book.' When I showed it to my professor, the feedback I received was, 'Your idea and choice of medium are skillfully meshed, but your work is lacking the human connection. It needs stories of real people who are dealing with the disease.'

"So I began looking for ways to meet women with breast cancer who might share with me what they were going through."

Understanding that some might be reluctant to talk about their illness, Cynthia went to the Breast Cancer Coalition's fall conference and approached Anne Weiher, the president of the coalition, with her idea and dilemma. Besides serving as the coalition's coordinator, Anne was also a psychologist. She was sensitive to the issues Cynthia had raised. Anne suggested that Cynthia talk to the women at the conference about her project. In addition, she offered to call others to ask whether they'd be interested. Harriette was one of the women she called.

When Harriette said she was open to it, she really had no idea what Cynthia had in mind. She wasn't thinking of her participation as an act of advocacy; she just wanted to be helpful. She had no inkling of the powerful impact Cynthia's project would eventually have.

"I just wanted to impress Cynthia," Harriette told me later. "And when she came to visit, I told her about the Danskin Triathlon I'd just completed. I guess she was impressed, because she wanted to take some still shots of me. She asked if I would pose for the pictures at her studio in Boulder. 'Bring your running shoes, your biking gear, and your swimming gear,' she said. I didn't know what to expect, but Stanley and I drove up there for the photo shoot."

Cynthia took a whole roll of pictures of Harriette. Her intention was to transfer some of the photographs onto a quilt. She was going to dedicate this project to Lovey Meeker, her mother's best friend, who had passed away from breast cancer. Lovey had been diagnosed with breast cancer while Cynthia was an undergraduate student at the University of Iowa. Sadly, by the time Lovey's cancer was discovered it had already metastasized to her brain, and she passed away only one year after her diagnosis. It had a huge impact on Cynthia.

After she took the still photos of Harriette in her studio, Cynthia asked whether she could follow Harriette to her chemotherapy appointments. At the clinic she shot photos of the syringe, the IV pole, and Harriette's port. She wanted the photos on the quilt to tell Harriette's breast cancer story. "Later, Cynthia asked me if I would pose nude from the waist up," Harriette said. "I asked Stanley how he felt about me doing that, and he said, 'Do whatever you want,' so I did it."

Through Anne's connections, Cynthia interviewed other women besides Harriette and documented their stories onto quilts, too. Her project eventually evolved into nine velvet quilts featuring a number of women, including one quilt she named the Breast Cancer History Quilt. Cynthia believed that quilts were beautiful and seductive objects of comfort and a way for a woman to make her own mark in time. The juxtaposition she created with the Breast Cancer History Quilt was a blatant display of an ugly disease on something very soft. She described what she did in a statement she made to a magazine published by DePauw University:

> I have presented a patchwork of the history of breast cancer. Instead of chronicling the history in an academic manner, I have included varied references to give the viewer more of a sense of the history of the disease. The earliest extant medical documents of breast cancer appear in Egyptian papyri from the eighteenth dynasty, 1587–1328 B.C. The first successful mastectomy was in the 1700s and, since the accounts in the Egyptian papyri, only four advancements have been made towards the treatment of breast cancer: the mastectomy, chemotherapy, radiation and Tamoxifen, a drug-based hormone therapy.
>
> The central image of the history quilt is a computer generated image of Fanny Burney, an English novelist who wrote one of the first personal accounts of breast cancer, with her diary entries from her mastectomy in 1811 printed in red text over her portrait. The diary entry is horrific and in many ways impos-

sible to imagine. Fanny Burney endured her mastectomy without anesthesia. Her account is written at a time when it was very inappropriate for a woman, or anyone for that matter, to talk about breast cancer. Much like the women I have interviewed, she had told her story. Through the history quilt, I am addressing the timeless nature of breast cancer and the common assumption that cancer is a disease of the 20th century.[1]

Cynthia named her entire quilt project *common threads*, in reference to the women's scars and the thread used to stitch each of their bodies back together, and then the quilts went on display, first at the CU arts building in April 1998. Harriette's family attended the grand opening of *common threads*. "I'm not an emotional person, but when we walked into the gallery, I was unexpectedly overwhelmed," Harriette said. "The quilts are huge. One is seven by six feet and another is twelve by seven." Harriette knew all of the women featured on the quilts. Among them were Sonia Mueller, Peggy Miller, Lois Hjelmstad, and her good friend Vicki Tosher.

"Peggy's quilt shows her covering one bare breast with her hand," Harriette said. "Embroidered gold around the border of Peggy's quilt read: *My mother had only one breast to feed me on*. Sonia's quilt said: *I had never seen my Dad cry until I shaved my head after my chemo treatment*. And then there was me, naked, with my arms crossed over my chest in a defiant pose." Harriette was surprised Cynthia had chosen the nude photo for the main picture. The defiance made her look back into the past and remember the time she got into trouble in the fourth grade. "The teacher had pulled my hair and, when I told my mother, she got mad and went to the school. The teacher defended herself by telling my mother I was too defiant."

Strangers at the exhibit must have come to the same conclusion when they saw Harriette's quilt. She recalled one person who had recognized her on the quilt and had turned to her and said, "You'll never die; you're too defiant." "That made me feel good, and right then I regretted that I hadn't invited more people to come to the opening. I just didn't know how they would react to my posing nude."

Harriette laughed about it now, but when I asked whether she had cried when she first saw the quilts, she said, "No. I don't cry. But I hadn't expected them to be so spectacular."

As I knew Harriette so well now, the most powerful part of *common threads* for me was the gold lettering on her quilt, which read: *I will be on chemo for the rest of my life.*

After its grand opening in Boulder in the spring of 1998, common threads *traveled to be on display at DePauw University in Greencastle, Indiana, and at the Muscatine Art Center in Iowa. The following year it made a powerful statement at the Women's Physicians conference in Des Moines, Iowa, and at the Art Center in Galesburg, Illinois. Since then,* common threads *has sparked the emotions of many people in galleries across the United States, from Texas to Michigan to New York to Louisiana. Harriette became a national icon, representing each one of us in the sisterhood of breast cancer.*

CHAPTER 24

More Worries

It had been nine years since Harriette's cancer came back—nine years that she had been going to the Rocky Mountain Cancer Center *alone* for her chemotherapy. On a Friday in December 2001, I sat with her while her Aredia dripped. She'd gotten her chemotherapy two weeks previously and this time needed only the Aredia for her bones. Now, almost ten years since her recurrence, Harriette was reflecting on the cancer that had brought her to this clinic. She was still worrying about it and wondering whether she ever would have had breast cancer at all if she'd had had the hysterectomy when she had been forty.

"I always had hormonal problems: migraines, missed periods in the summer, and heavy bleeding," she said. "I'll always wonder about it."

Besides that, she had even more worries. She told me that Cyndi had recently been hospitalized for some gynecological problems and that she herself was having leg pain from slipping on some ice in Washington Park. Falling on her bad hip, she'd also banged the back of her head. She was still a little dizzy nearly a week later. "I was having a hard time this week walking down the stairs at Jeff's house with this radiating pain." With her lingering New York accent, she pronounced it like "sta-yuhs."

I often found it hard to keep up with Harriette as she bounced from subject to subject but found it more difficult when she seemed overly stressed. She said she was behind on the financial reports for her son's fertilizer business that she was supposed to have ready for the accountant, and she was anxious, waiting for Stanley's new insurance to kick in, because he had some basal cell carcinoma he needed taken care of, and he needed some heart tests done, too. Harriette was worrying about problems with her own insurance and fussing about having to pay $178 a month for it while possibly having to pay full cost for all of her medications if they were not going to be covered by Medicare. She was also worried about Cyndi's continuing weight loss. "She's down to one hundred pounds," Harriette said. On top of all of that, with this being the end of Hanukkah, Harriette was having a party at their house the next afternoon. She was planning to cook some traditional foods: brisket and applesauce, chicken breasts, and potato latkes.

Harriette had so many problems I couldn't keep up with all of them. There was really nothing I could do other than listen. Sometimes listening was the best thing to do anyway. I found when people listened to me I could usually sort out problems myself, and afterward they didn't feel so big.

After Harriette got everything off her chest, she put her lounge chair back and covered herself, pulling a blanket over her chic black pants. She said the IV drip made her cold sometimes. Her feet, in two-inch heeled black-tie shoes, hung out from the end of the blanket. With the calming effect of the Aredia drip, she nodded off a couple of times while we were talking. Finally, I said, "I'd better let you nap now. You're exhausted."

A month later, on January 11, 2002, she looked calm in the afternoon when we met at the Cancer Center. As we followed the oncology nurse to a private room, Harriette seemed different. She was not her normal hyper-self, and I suspected something had happened. Then she told me.

"I'll only be coming once a month from now on," she said. "I found out on Monday that the chemo has stopped working. I haven't told Cyndi, but I'm on Arimidex now—one pill a day."

Her dumb tumors had become smart. After ten years they had become resistant to the 5-FU that Dr. Garfield had prescribed. Because he had since retired, Harriette's new oncologist would have to change her treatment. The next step was to try the hormones again. Fortunately for Harriette, there was now Arimidex, an aromatase inhibitor. Aromatase is an enzyme in muscles, fat, and the liver that can turn the hormone androgen into estrogen. Arimidex blocks the process so this estrogen cannot feed the tumors. The new drug had been approved by the FDA in 2000 after trials and had shown it was more effective than tamoxifen in lowering the body's estrogen to cut off the breast cancer cells' nutritional source.[1]

"Dr. Hinshaw noticed me limping the last time she saw me in December," Harriette said. "So she ordered a bone scan, and then she wanted a tumor marker test."

Since July, Harriette had already been having these blood tests every three months to monitor the biomarkers, CA 27–29. These proteins are in everyone's blood; however, in breast cancer, when there is metastasis to the bones, they're found in increased amounts. Dr. Hinshaw wanted to determine whether Harriette's markers had gone up. "She called and said that my markers had gone up two hundred points," Harriette told me. That indicated new tumor activity. "She kept asking me over the phone, 'Are you sure you're not in pain?'" Dr. Hinshaw was going to show Harriette her bone scan that day.

I watched the oncology nurse expertly draw blood from Harriette's port and begin the line for the Aredia. While the two of them chatted back and forth, I silently worried what this all meant for her. "I need another job to pay for the medicine," Harriette told the nurse with a nervous laugh. Harriette admitted she felt leery about the effectiveness of the new hormone drug, Arimidex, since tamoxifen hadn't worked for her in 1992.

"Maybe your body's just ready for something new," the nurse said lightheartedly.

"Well, I've been sleeping pretty well lately because Cyndi's been in the hospital," Harriette said. The reason she'd been sleeping well was not because she wasn't worried. It was because she hadn't had to get up with Cyndi during the nights. Harriette actually had a host of worries. "Cyndi has pancreatitis," she said. "She's down to 85 pounds. We're crushing her pills now and putting them in applesauce because she's having trouble swallowing. She's saying, 'Mom, I'm losing control.' I can't find a doctor who will take her. Nobody will take Medicare. She's so sick they don't know what to do with her. Then, I was opening my mail at eleven o'clock last night, and a letter from the Social Security Administration informed me they're reviewing my disability status. I don't know what I'll do if I don't get disability." A single-pill-a-day of Arimidex costs $229 a month. Harriette told us her Aredia cost $1,800 a month. Cyndi was on the same medicine for her bones, too.

The only good news Harriette had to share was that she was going to England soon with Jeff. "I never thought I'd go to Europe. This is a spur-of-the-moment thing for us. We've always planned our trips years in advance." Jeff had surprised her with this trip. It was a thank-you gift for all the help she gave him with his business.

Harriette had worried herself nearly sick while he had been in the hospital, and she was spread thin between tending to Cyndi at home, standing by Jeff's side, and driving Stanley to the hospital for his heart tests. Still, she had managed to make it to her chemotherapy appointments on time.

Soon, Harriette was on the phone answering a page from Stanley. It seemed like she was always answering pages when we were together. "Don't stop at the pharmacy. Get her into the house," she was saying. "She'll have to slide off onto the couch by herself. Drive careful with her." Stanley was driving Cyndi home from the hospital. Before she hung up the phone, Harriette reminded him to buy some sourdough bread and applesauce for Cyndi.

"He's had an angiogram recently, and he's not supposed to lift over fifteen pounds," she told me. "He can't transfer her. We're both scared right now. Stanley's so nervous, he's forgetting things."

Harriette continued talking while I was getting more concerned about her. It was as if she were just talking out loud to herself. "I'm so afraid that I'll get sick and lose my hair. Now, I'm going to have to find a way to tell Cyndi because everybody else knows—though, I really don't have to because nothing's really changed. I just have new medicine."

By now, Harriette had the chair in the laid-back position. She tossed and turned from side to side, trying to find a comfortable position for her painful right hip. "I start physical therapy tomorrow. We don't know what this is. Maybe it's sciatica from my fall on the ice in Washington Park last month."

She told me that another time, shortly after her fall in the park, she had suddenly jammed her toe when she kicked something hard hidden under the snow. "I couldn't put any pressure on my leg after that. Or maybe I have a tumor that's sitting on a nerve. This pain is worse than what I had in '98," she said.

Harriette was upset because she wasn't able to do the lunges and squats in her exercise routine. "It kills my hip, and I can't increase the weight, and I can't do body pumps or the bike spinning class." But nothing had showed up on the recent X-ray of her hip that could explain the pain.

The bone scan showed a different story, however. The white spots of tumor activity were on the spine and the left hip—different places from where the pain was now. The doctor thought perhaps it was referred pain.

Harriette found out the Arimidex had side effects, too, such as aches from the flu and muscle weakness. "I've already had to reduce my bike riding speed because I don't feel too well," she said. "I was worried about riding outside, and Jeff said, 'Don't worry, Mom, we'll get you a better bike.'"

I knew I might hear this news from Harriette one day about the chemo not working anymore, but I didn't expect it to come so soon in our relationship. I was concerned about her and told her so. "I think you've done so well all this time because you had to, for Cyndi. But, there *are* new drugs, so you never know. I'm glad to hear you're going to England."

She asked me whether my first book was published yet. I told her I was looking for a publisher, and she smiled. Harriette had stopped tossing and turning and lay comfortable finally, with a blanket spread over her black corduroy pants. Where the nurse had laid back the black velvet collar of Harriette's red print blouse, I could see her port pouched beneath her skin.

"I'm honored that you're writing about me," Harriette said. She paused for a beat and said, "I'm reevaluating my life. I've got to decide how I want to spend my time now. I've thought about all the things that add the most substance to my life and which things I might be willing to eliminate. I'm still tutoring, but recently I got four calls to do Reach to Recovery visits. I need to break from that right now. I'm too distraught to be trying to cheer up other people."

Harriette confided that she'd had a "flash" about having this recurrence. It came the previous summer when some friends suggested she train for another triathlon to celebrate her sixtieth birthday. "I remembered that I got my first recurrence while I was training for the triathlon to celebrate my fiftieth birthday. After my friends said that, I had a premonition about this one."

Harriette didn't want to stop any of her other activities, though. She was bummed that she'd lost out on a friend's generous email offer of free tickets to see the play *Tommy*. Because she had so much on her mind, she'd overlooked reading the email.

I called Harriette a few weeks later because I knew she was soon leaving for her trip to England. She was packing and complaining about muscle aches that were hampering her progress. "The aches are a side effect of the Arimidex, and this persistent sciatica," she rationalized. "I'm excited to go to England," she said, "but not looking forward to ten hours on the plane with sciatica. It's good I have an aisle seat."

Cyndi had just been released from the hospital after her bout with pancreatitis, followed by a pulmonary complication. Harriette was wearing a mask around the house to keep from infecting Cyndi with anything more. It was for both of their benefit. In her dogged determination, she didn't want anything to disrupt her and Jeff's departure.

CHAPTER 25

Menopause at Twenty-eight

The more I came to know Harriette, the more inspired I was by how she never let obstacles stand in her way. I noticed her influence on me, in subtle ways every day. On afternoon walks, when I began to tire plugging uphill, I would think of Harriette and push myself a little farther, to get to the top of Conifer Mountain. I started doing pushups—only a couple at first, but then added more like I imagined Harriette would do. If I went swimming, I would swim one or two laps more after I was ready to quit, like I knew Harriette would do.

Harriette was never far from my thoughts, but while she was away, I got a chance to get together with Kim. We didn't get together very often, and I hadn't seen her in several months, but I liked keeping in touch with her. I treasured my new breast cancer friends, young and old. Kim was my youngest breast cancer friend. Since Kim and I both liked Starbucks, we met there.

It was cool and overcast in late January, and Kim was already sipping her coffee when I got there. "I just came from having my blood drawn," she said. It was her routine check for tumor markers. After Kim's treatment for an aggressive, invasive breast cancer, her oncologist kept a vigilant surveillance on her. "It always makes me nervous getting my blood tests," she said.

Although these tests are not always accurate, nor very useful in detecting early breast cancer, if a protein called CEA (carcinoembryonic antigen) was elevated in her blood, it could be a sign of an active tumor, a metastasis. Kim would hear back from her doctor if there was anything to worry about.

"I hope it comes out all right," I said. "I'm due for a mammogram, and I'm a little nervous myself." No matter how young or healthy we are, after cancer we can never feel like we are totally out of the woods.

Although it had been three years since Kim's diagnosis, her doctors were still following her closely. That was comforting, but as a young survivor, she did have one complaint I didn't. "My doctor insists that I have yearly mammograms. I'm still young, and it seems like I'm subjecting myself to too much radiation. It's all cumulative," she said. She didn't know whether she felt any comfort from her doctor's reassurances that the amount of radiation in one mammogram was equal to the amount a person acquires on one airplane trip. She reasoned, "If I don't have a mammogram, that's one more plane trip I can take instead!"

Kim looked forward to her trips. She had recently been to Barbados, where the weather had been warm and beautiful and the water crystal blue. "I needed that vacation," she said. "I had so much work in November and December that I'd nearly fallen into the loony bin."

She was leading a normal, hectic life. Nevertheless, it remained difficult not to worry about the long-term side effects—something that might occur later on as a result of her cancer treatment. She still had a whole life ahead of her.

"I'm glad I had chemotherapy," she said. "I know I had to, but I'm not so glad I had the radiation. I try not to think too much about the effects it might have had on my heart and my bones and ribs."

Even though Kim had no regrets about the chemotherapy now, looking back on her treatments was still emotional for her. "The AC was especially hard. First, I had to go for outpatient surgery to have a port put in." Pulling back on its lapel, she opened her black leather jacket and showed me the small scar on the inside of her upper arm, a reminder of where it had been. "Then, I went for my first treatment."

Only Kim's mother had come with her to the Cancer Center that day. "My dad just couldn't do it," Kim said. "Mom told me that while we were waiting for the nurse to bring me the release forms. Even I had had to do a lot of self-talk to get myself there. I could hardly believe that I'd agreed to take poisonous chemicals into my body. I said to Mom, 'I could just walk out now and not do this.'"

Instead, Kim had busied herself with the release form while the nurse prepared the bags of chemicals and the IV tubing that would drip them through the port. The form described risks and possible side effects, including the warning that chemotherapy could put a young woman into premature menopause—something Kim hadn't come across in her prior research. It was a possible side effect of the Cytoxan, the alkylating agent that attacked rapidly dividing cells, including egg cells. "No one had mentioned this to me," Kim said. "I was still young, only twenty-eight. What if I wanted children some day? Hadn't my doctor considered that?"

Since breast cancer occurred only in approximately one out of two thousand women in Kim's age group, it was as though everyone had overlooked the ramifications it had on young women who still had dreams of marriage and children.[1] "I was devastated," Kim said. "I'd already made up my mind to do the chemotherapy and then, so abruptly, I was learning that maybe I would never have children." Kim brought her fingers up to catch the tears suddenly spilling from her eyes.

Seeing her emotion stirred my own, and my eyes filled up, too. Wiping hers, she said, "Mom cried that day, too, but she kept smiling, and she said, 'It'll be okay.'

"Then my doctor reassured me that there was only a ten percent chance that the chemotherapy would cause permanent menopause in a woman my age. He always had an answer for my questions. He had a reputation for being one of the best in Denver, and he had the attitude that none of his patients would die from breast cancer. His self-assured manner made me trust him. I took the ten percent chance and decided not to worry. I thought worrying about it would just work against me."

Not knowing what to expect after the first treatment, Kim and her mother stopped at the pharmacy for anti-nausea medicine and then headed straight to Kim's townhouse. "It took several drugs to control the nausea over the next few days, and the drugs made me sleepy. I wasn't really sick, but I didn't feel quite right either. I just ate to try to feel better."

The next week, the father of the guy she was dating passed away from lung cancer. "I'd only known his father for a short time. Since I met him shortly after my own diagnosis, it made it especially difficult watching him decline."

At his funeral in her hometown of Pueblo, she saw some of her friends but didn't speak to any of them about her cancer. "In such a small town as Pueblo, almost everyone knows each other, and I didn't want people talking about me. I didn't want to risk upsetting my boyfriend any more than he already was. It was easy to hide my cancer anyway, since I'd only had one chemotherapy treatment. I still had my hair."

Three weeks later it was time again for her next treatment. "My appointments were always on Fridays," Kim said. "And the Monday before, I would always start getting tremendous anxiety. I just didn't want to go and do it again. I was working forty hours a week and freelancing too. I was exhausted and often went to bed by eight o'clock."

After the second treatment her shoulder-length hair started falling out, as did the rest of her body hair. It was a side effect of the Adriamycin. "It happened *two weeks to the day* of when I was told it would. People at work started finding strands of it everywhere, even before I noticed it. Then I called an old friend of mine and asked him to come over and cut my hair because I knew he had some clippers. He buzzed off all the rest of my hair. It was harder on him than me because I was prepared for it, but I still got upset seeing all of my hair in the trashcan. I couldn't throw it away for a while." Kim kept the hair in the trashcan for a month.

"I got a wig of my same color and style and wore it to work. It was hot and itchy, so I usually took it off after I got there. Once, I forgot to wear it when I went out, and people stared at me with dirty looks. It was like they were saying, *why did you do that to your hair?* The wig was a nuisance and, one time, I accidentally singed it when I was cooking. I had to cut it to make it look right again."

Kim found out that she really didn't mind being bald. "I was just too fatigued to care. I was going to aerobics classes, trying to keep strong, and I wore a hat that had a false tuft of hair sticking out, that I tied into a bun. But the AC finally knocked me on my butt, and I stopped doing the aerobics class altogether."

The AC also caused weird little skin tags to grow on her face and made her eyes swollen some days. Her menstrual periods stopped, and she was bothered by severe hot flashes every half hour. Mostly, she was mentally exhausted trying to live a normal life and deal with cancer at the same time. "People from work would give me pep talks, saying I was going to be okay, and I told myself that I just had to make it to the Taxol cycle, which would be much easier. I wasn't exercising anymore, but before each chemotherapy treatment, I did get onto my Stair Master. I pumped the steps like it was my war dance." Kim never told anyone she frequently thought about quitting the treatments, but she never did miss an appointment. She was always back to work on the following Monday.

Along with the Taxol treatments came pain in her jaw and other joints. The pain in her hips and knees made it difficult to walk after the first week. Though the drug had uncomfortable side effects, it was necessary following the AC. Taxol hit the cancer cells at a different stage of division than the AC. It was this combination of drugs that made the chemotherapy more effective. Fortunately for Kim, a week of Advil, muscle relaxants, and Glucosamine Chondroitin had her walking again without the pain.

Then there was the mysterious Sunday pain in her teeth. "They hurt all over and inside as if acid was eating through them, like I'd eaten too many oranges. The pain kept recurring, and it always happened on Sundays." Eventually Kim realized it was on the Sundays following the Friday Taxol treatments. Last, she lost the hair on her legs, which for some reason hadn't come off during the AC.

As if she hadn't been beaten up enough, the final straw was when her boyfriend told her he didn't want to see her anymore. "He said he just couldn't deal with cancer again. I noticed a few of my other friends weren't coming around anymore either, but others who I never would have expected, were there for me."

Although it was an emotionally difficult time, Kim found solace at work and at the Cancer Center, where all the other patients were there for breast cancer, too. "It was like a party most of the time. There was plenty of food, and we could talk about our experiences together. That helped me, and eventually I became stronger in dealing with my cancer alone."

Taking chemotherapy was tough, but Kim thought she had tolerated it well since she hadn't suffered any infections. "My white blood cell count never dropped below 2,400," she boasted, "compared to my friends, whose counts had dropped below 500. Five to ten thousand is considered normal," she said. "And when I was completely done with my treatment, I felt strong again quickly. It was strange because three weeks after my last treatment, my count was already up to 7,500. My cells had never been more than 4,500 during all of the other three-week intervals. It was as if my body knew it was over and was jubilant."

"I can't remember the date I started chemotherapy, but I remember the day I completed it. July 16th," she proclaimed. "Mentally, I was feeling great, and my hair was coming back in very fine and curly blond patches. I'd never been blond, so later, when I had enough hair, I dyed it dark brown. My new short hair became my strength and confidence."

I smiled at Kim's confidence and told her from now on I would always celebrate her recovery on July 16th. It was a special day for me, too. It was my birthday. Besides breast cancer, we had something else in common.

Another day, over dessert at Cucina Colore, Kim told me about her experience with radiation treatments, which reminded me of my reticence early on, when I thought I might have to undergo radiation. When I chose the mastectomy, radiation became a non-issue for me, yet I saw others shared my misgivings about the treatment. Now that I'd learned more about it, I didn't have the same fear as before, but I understood Kim's feelings very well.

Her radiation began three weeks after she completed chemotherapy. "I remember not feeling very confident with my radiation oncologists," she said. "I had two doctors, and they couldn't tell me if I should have five weeks or six weeks of radiation. They seemed so wishy-washy. I wish now that I'd researched more about radiation, but, at that time, I was feeling so elated that the chemotherapy was over, I just went ahead with it.

"The whole six weeks was sort of a blur. I would go there early every morning and was in and out in just a few minutes." Initially, her only side effect from the radiation was a light burn on her skin. "That showed up fairly soon. The nurses gave me lotions to take care of the burn. Then, about half way through the six weeks, I noticed my breast hurting. It was a deep ache that spread up and over my shoulder. They said it wasn't normal to feel that kind of pain, so I worried they were doing something wrong. I learned later from talking with other women that they experienced this, too."

Kim said she still had a pain in her scapula three years later, and she blamed it on the radiation. But the burn to her skin from radiation was nothing compared to the blow of chemotherapy. "Chemotherapy took me down physically and mentally. It took energy to keep talking myself through the treatments, but I knew I had to have the chemotherapy. I just regret I had radiation. Of course, my radiation was three years ago, and things have probably changed already," Kim said.

One of her friends had had radiation recently, after receiving several consultations, including one at the Mayo Clinic. "Hers was a modified treatment that limits penetration in a more controlled fashion. She told me that the medical people here didn't even know what 'modified treatment' she was talking about."

Kim wished she could have had that modified treatment. "I'm young, and I don't think there's been enough study on young women to know what kind of side effects might show up twenty years later. My doctor said the effects of radiation are most damaging to people younger than thirty."

Kim remained frightened about what might be in her future. "Maybe I'll get cancer in my ribs later." In the meantime she was arming herself with a handful of nuts every day, almonds mostly—to knock out cancer.

A lot of things about chemotherapy and radiation worried Kim, yet she stayed optimistic about her ovaries. She never let herself believe she would be in the ten percent of young women who would become menopausal from the chemotherapy. "I had terribly annoying hot flashes every day from chemotherapy," Kim said. "And then one day about four weeks after my radiation stopped, I experienced pain in my abdomen. A few days later, my period started." It was truly something to celebrate, and then the hot flashes disappeared, too.

Strangely, one year after chemotherapy had ended, Kim said the weird skin tags reappeared on her face. Her eyes became swollen and bothersome, and her eyelashes fell out again. Soon after came the annoying pain in her teeth. "I realized my cells had memory, and they were just re-experiencing the effects of chemotherapy." Luckily, the effects subsided in a few days. Now all the side effects seemed worth it. She had a whole life left to live.

CHAPTER 26

Chemobrain

> God put me on earth to accomplish a certain number of things.
> Right now, I am so far behind, I will never die.
> I remember when I remembered, when I was organized, when information stayed in my head, and when my analytical skills were strong...
> Harriette Grober, *May 12, 2001, Day of Caring*

Looking back, I remembered Harriette, one month after I first met her. She was sitting on stage with a panel of women. Before her was a room full of participants at the Day of Caring. She wore a black-and-white dress with nylon stockings and heels. I've never seen her in a dress since, but that day was special because she was addressing the audience with her personal story. It was related to the side effects of her chemotherapy and difficulties she experienced with cognition in 1997. The "difficulties" she was talking about were something we didn't have a name for at the time she was experiencing them, but now it's become recognized as a phenomenon called chemobrain.

Among her rapt listeners in the audience was me, hearing about chemobrain for the first time. I was learning a lot that day about the disease whose ranks I had just joined, but, unlike others in the audience, I hadn't taken chemotherapy. This was a totally new topic for me. Some had described chemobrain as "a smorgasbord of neuropsychological impairments resulting from treatment with chemotherapy." The symptoms of memory loss, language difficulties, and problems in concentration, including loss of the ability to multitask, seem to vary in individuals from negligible to severe.[1] And because women have been complaining to their doctors about these vague symptoms for so long, neuropsychologists were finally looking into chemobrain as a valid and true phenomenon. The panel members who were familiar with chemobrain described what it was like for them, but it was Harriette's story that captured me. It enabled me to understand what living with it must be like.

"My job had been my life," Harriette said. "I was not one of those people who would have said they should have spent less time at the office. I could juggle ten things at once and not drop a single ball. But after three years on chemotherapy, the juggler began to fall apart, and the balls started dropping one by one. At first I refused to acknowledge that I could no longer do it all. For two more years I tried harder and harder to remain skilled and proficient, yet I was becoming increasingly disorganized. I was forgetting deadlines and making scheduling mistakes.

"Where I used to be a computer whiz, remembered all the shortcuts, and picked up new skills quickly, I was starting to have difficulty learning how to use the new programs. It was both humiliating and frustrating. And then, I experienced a flash."

Harriette often talked of premonitions she'd had. When she spoke of one in particular, she called it "a flash." In this flash she told the audience that she saw herself losing her job because things were not going well. "For some time, my chair at work had felt very uncomfortable, but I feared if I asked for a new one, my boss might say no because she would be thinking that I would be leaving soon. Finally, I asked for a new chair anyway and was surprised when she said, 'Sure.' However, not long after, it became clear that it would be better for everyone if I stopped working. Sadly, I resigned from the job I loved."

The loss caused her to slip into a depression that created further problems in the family when she couldn't make decisions. She kept changing her mind about things she thought they should buy or things she felt they couldn't buy, and she often found herself angry and yelling. She would shout at them, things like, "If I'm lucky, I'll die from this!" Antidepressant medication didn't help. It caused her to feel like she was jumping out of her skin. Eventually, she found herbal supplements to help curb the turbulence of her depression.

"In 1997, when my employer and I decided it would be mutually beneficial if I retired, it was the biggest loss of my life," Harriette confided. "But over time I've learned to accept the changes in my life and the person I am now. It's taken me almost four years to get to this point. I went through a severe depression to where I lost my appetite and had difficulty sleeping. I suffered from debilitating migraine headaches. When I had always been the one in the group at the restaurant who could figure out each person's share of the bill in my head, I was resorting to pencil and paper. Realizing my brain wasn't working the way it used to, I was scared."

After some deep searching spiritually, Harriette recognized that she was more than her job title or her body parts. "Where I used to compete in swimming and amateur Volvo tennis, I now enjoy helping my son with his seasonal business and look forward to our bike rides on nice days," she said.

"My daughter and I have survived many tough times together, and now we boost our spirits with our motto, *When the going gets tough, the tough get tougher*. We enjoy our favorite song, 'You Are the Wind Beneath My Wings.'"

Although much had changed in her life because of chemobrain, some things were no different. "The love I have for my family and friends and the need I have to exercise every day haven't changed. Without these two constants in my life, I believe I wouldn't be here today. Most importantly, though, two members of the family, an affenpinscher and cock-a-poo, never noticed that I changed at all."

A certain grace and comfort with her cancer shone through in Harriette's attitude. "The first grader whom I tutor is beginning to read chapter books now. Well, the cancer has provided me a different chapter in my life, and that's all right. But, with everything, there comes a price. In retrospect, the price of chemobrain is cheap compared to the alternative I face without chemotherapy. I'm glad to be alive, and I'm learning to take the time to smell the roses.

"I feel privileged to be able to share my coping strategies for chemobrain. Some people may be upset to know that chemobrain is a reality; however, for me, it was a comfort to know that it's real, and I couldn't have done anything to prevent the balls from falling. Research has shown that chemotherapy causes fatigue and anemia in some patients. Now, it's important that more research be done to prove the validity of our complaints of chemobrain."

Harriette received a hearty applause after she recited this parable she'd read in a swimming magazine. It seemed to typify her:

Two frogs fell into a deep cream bowl
One was an optimistic soul.
But the other took the gloomy view.
"We'll drown," he cried, without much ado,
and with a lasting despairing cry,
he flung up his legs and said,
"Good-bye."

Quote the other frog with a steadfast grin,
"I can't get out, but I won't give in.
I'll just swim around till my strength is spent,
Then I'll die the more content."

Bravely he swam to work his scheme,
and his struggles began to churn the cream.
The more he swam, his legs a flutter,
the more the cream turned into butter.

On top of the butter at last he stopped
And out of the bowl he gaily hopped.
What is the moral? It's easily found.
It you can't hop out, keep swimming around!

Author Unknown

CHAPTER 27

Arimidex or Taxotere?

Driving to the Cancer Center, it felt a little too warm for the eighth of February. The groundhog had seen his shadow, which meant we were supposed to have six more weeks of winter. Although we'd had intermittent cold snaps, it seemed we hadn't had much of a winter yet, with so little snow. This kind of weather wasn't normal for Colorado. I remembered growing up in Denver when we often had dumps of two and three feet of snow and enough cold that we made ice skating rinks with the hose in our backyard. Years later, after Jim and I got married and built our house on Conifer Mountain, it was not uncommon for him to spend hours shoveling five to six feet of snow off the roof on the north side of our house. Maybe we would still get some snow this season. We sure needed it.

I was anxious to see Harriette after her return from England. She was on the phone in the lobby of the Cancer Center when I arrived, pre-registering her daughter for oral surgery. "I just saw the doctor," she said when she hung up. "I don't think the Arimidex is working." She looked tired and drained, different than I'd seen her before, and it worried me.

We started toward the treatment area, and I could see she was limping. "I still have the same pain in my hips," she said. She was in a hurry to get her Aredia drip going. She had a physical therapy appointment afterward. "If the Arimidex doesn't work, the doctor said we'll have to try Taxotere next. I don't know anyone who's lasted more than two years on that."

Harriette knew that Taxotere meant she was moving down the line of agents for breast cancers that didn't respond to hormones or other chemotherapies. Taxotere attacks the cancer cells by interfering with their ability to divide, so they're unable to grow. It also attacks white blood cells, which would leave her susceptible to infections. If she started this drug, she would get it in a one-hour infusion, every three weeks. "I'm going to lose my hair, and I'll have to tell Cyndi," she said. She hadn't informed her daughter of the new development in her cancer, and she was worried how Cyndi would take it.

In spite of the pain in her hip, Harriette said she and Jeff had managed to see five plays and visit several museums in London. "We're like two peas in a pod. We both love the health and science museums. We walked everywhere, and I lost weight because the food was so expensive. We hardly ate."

I watched the nurse draw Harriette's blood from the port. They were going to check her tumor markers again. The last time they were checked, her CEA had increased, and the CA 27-29 number had been close to six hundred. The normal numbers for the CA 27-29 proteins are between zero and thirty. "In a few weeks I'll have scans to see if they show any more tumor growth," Harriette told me. Then they would decide about Taxotere. The thought of it weighed heavily.

Just as Harriette's treatment options seemed to be drying up, so was Colorado. With so little precipitation, we were entering a troublesome drought situation. It was forbidding, but finally, after one month, there were some things to celebrate. Snow was falling, and the Arimidex was working. The first flakes became visible just as Harriette and I each pulled up to the Cancer Center, where she was coming for her first monthly $2,227 IV infusion of Zometa. She was switching over to Zometa and hoped that the new pricey medicine would work as well as the Aredia had to protect her bones from the malignancy.

As we walked toward the building, Harriette told me she had started and discontinued chemotherapy again. "I had one treatment and then stopped because my hip is much better," she remarked. "I know the hormones are working on the tumors now."

This was good news, and still there was more to celebrate. Birthdays. A lot of people hate them because birthdays mean they're getting older. People dread the physical decline that comes with aging. But after cancer, we're grateful for birthdays. They're a gift. They mean we're alive. Both Harriette and Cyndi had birthdays this month. Cyndi would turn thirty-seven and Harriette sixty. Harriette said she was looking forward to the weekend because she was going to Heritage Square, a tourist and shopping area near the foothills, to try out a new bike—a birthday present that weighed twenty-three pounds. "It's lighter than my old one and resistant to flats and blowouts," she boasted.

"Can you still try out the bike if it's snowing?" I asked.

"I don't know," she said. "I'm afraid of the ice."

Then Harriette informed me they were living in a hotel. "We've been there for three weeks. We had to get out of our house because we discovered a mold problem in the kitchen." The mold came from a long-term undetected leak from the refrigerator's icemaker that had been seeping under the floor until the linoleum had finally become mushy. "The floor was so uneven I was scared it would collapse and cause Cyndi to spill out of her wheelchair. She'd fall down into the crawl space."

They realized that the mold had been contributing to some of Cyndi's illnesses for a long time. The insurance company was not only paying to replace the cabinets and the floor, but was also footing the bill for a luxury suite at the hotel where they got their room cleaned every day, their sheets changed, complimentary breakfasts, and warm homemade cookies in the afternoons. Sometimes even dinner snacks with wine and beer were provided free.

Though Harriette was happy about some of these things, she was clearly upset about others, one of which gave me cause to worry. "I'm short of breath," she said. "I notice it when I'm walking the dogs or working out. I called the nurse to tell her about it, and she asked me if I wanted oxygen. I told her no."

But Harriette wanted the nurse to check her oxygen level before she received her IV medication. Since she only had the problem when she was exercising, we hurried to the stairs to walk up and down a few flights first. Since she was a seasoned athlete, I hoped I could keep up with her. She actually tired first, running short of breath before I did.

Harriette's pulse-ox checked out normal. "Ninety-five percent," the nurse said. Holding a needle in her hand, the nurse asked her, as if she didn't know, "Where's your port, my dear?" Harriette nonchalantly opened her blouse and took a deep breath as the nurse pressed the needle into the port.

"Is everybody switched over to Zometa now?" Harriette asked.

"Many of them have."

A lot of doctors were substituting Zometa for Aredia. The new bisphosphonate drug had been specifically developed for cancer patients, unlike Aredia, which was originally developed for treating osteoporosis. Since Zometa works similarly to Aredia in inhibiting bone resorption, it's preferred because it's more powerful and can be administered in fifteen minutes—a lot more quickly than Aredia. If it were infused any more quickly than fifteen minutes, it would prove too toxic for the kidneys and elevate the risk of renal failure.[1] Harriette's blood would have to be checked at each visit to monitor her kidneys.

From the picture window at the Cancer Center, we suddenly became aware that everything outside was covered in white. The snow was flying fiercely in a northerly direction. We hadn't seen weather like this all winter. We needed the moisture so badly, it was awesome, but it was also an hour commute home for me—in good weather. I feared what my trip was going to be like. "It looks like a blizzard," I said. "Maybe I should get going."

The weather concerned Harriette, too. She had several errands yet to do. "I have to get applesauce for Cyndi," she said.

I prepared to leave while she was still, unfortunately, hooked up to the IV. I told her on my way out, "We're going to celebrate your sixtieth birthday in two weeks. We'll have lunch at your favorite restaurant."

"The Fresh Fish Company," she hollered after me. As for the blizzard, the roads had quickly turned to ice in the city, and traffic was snarled badly. I wormed my way through and found there was hardly any snow west of the city. Harriette called me later. "It took me four hours to get home!" she said, wondering about me.

"It was nothing," I said. The blizzard had fizzled out.

CHAPTER 28

Grateful for Birthdays

———◆———

In April there was more cause for celebration. The cherry trees along Union Boulevard were in full bloom near my friend Pat's house. Whereas the other trees were still barren this early in the spring, their sweet scent drew my attention as I turned down the street to her house. Just like the trees, I found Pat in full bloom, all recovered now, and she was also feeling grateful for birthdays.

"All of last year I didn't do much of anything," she began as we settled in her living room. "But now, I'm back doing everything again. I'm happy to be alive—happy for every day I have. I'm not like I was on my sixtieth birthday." She laughed, remembering the day. "I bawled all day. Tried everything not to turn sixty. My boys were gone, and only my daughter Julie was at home. She and my husband Ray had a big birthday cake for me, and I wouldn't even look at it. I told them, 'I will have days, but not birthdays.'"

Now Pat reflected on the past year. "There were times when I was so sick, I thought, *Why doesn't God just take me? I don't want to be a sickly person.* My mother had been like that. She had every ache and pain imaginable, and ever since I was a child my father and I catered to her. She never did anything for herself—never shopped or cleaned. She wouldn't even turn a roast by herself. My father had to come home from work to do it for her.

"After my father died from cancer, my mother came to live with us, and I was still catering to her every whim. She called my daughter Julie, 'that girl.' It upset Julie so much that once when she was in high school working on a homecoming float she said, 'Mom, I'm leaving and not coming home.' Ray understood why. He said, 'She doesn't have a mother, and I don't have a wife.'"

Later, after Pat's doctor convinced her she had to put her mother into a nursing home, Pat visited her mother every day. "The staff could hear my mother nagging, and finally they would say it was time for me to go home."

Pat's mother passed away after complications from a fall, and now Pat was determined never to be like her mother. "When I was experiencing the bad effects of chemotherapy, I would think of how my mother complained so, and I would say, 'I have breast cancer, and there's nothing I can do to change that, but I won't give in to this pain.' Then I pushed myself to get better. My husband doesn't get sucked into complaining tactics anyway, so somehow all of that helped me cope with the breast cancer."

Since September 11th, I told Pat I'd spent time thinking about tragedies, big and small, and since we were speaking about coping, I asked her what she'd thought about during the day of September 11th, when the World Trade Center and the Pentagon were attacked. "I was eating breakfast when I saw the burning building on TV," she said. "I felt the very same horror in the pit of my stomach as when I heard on the radio that World War II had started. Like all Americans, I was down and dazed. I couldn't stay away from the news. I didn't even think about my breast cancer or myself that day. I know cancer is bad and mine can come back again, but there are treatments available to me. There are other things on earth that are so much worse."

I agreed. There are things worse than cancer.

CHAPTER 29

Peau d'Orange—A Bad Sign

Since November I'd been looking forward to getting together with my neighbor, Sue Niksic. We'd made arrangements several times, yet each time she'd had to cancel. Now it was April 24th, and at four o'clock in the afternoon, she called to cancel again. Between a full-time job, two active children, and organizing a sock hop benefit, she said, "There just never seems to be enough time. I find myself taking on too much, most of the time. I shouldn't do it because I get too tired."

I told her I understood. Sue explained that she was organizing the sock hop to raise funds for Ernie Krehl, the long-time school bus driver for our kids on Conifer Mountain. Ernie was in treatment for lung cancer, and the money was to help offset his medical expenses. "When I was sick, I had a hard time accepting people's help," she said, "but I needed it. Then after I got better, I decided to give back when I could by helping others who need it. My kids love Ernie. Maybe your kids remember him?"

"Yes, they do." Kids loved Ernie because he gave them treats and had fun with them while he kept them orderly on the bus. My son Matt said Ernie was in a good mood every day, and he wasn't mean to them like some bus drivers. Heather remembered that Ernie waved to everyone he passed on the road. She thought it was cool that after she got her driver's license, Ernie always waved to her when she drove by his bus. She felt good knowing he remembered her. Ernie was well known in the community also for his involvement with the Mountain Man Rendezvous, a group of history buffs who reenact the pioneer days at summer events across the state. My kids remembered Ernie giving Mountain Man demonstrations at their school.

Sue said her parents and sister had been demanding a lot of her time lately as well, and that she was planning to record some songs over the weekend with a friend.

"You sing?" I asked.

"Yes. I've done some singing; I used to do more."

I remembered how it was for me, working, when my kids were young and active in sports. I understood why she usually had to cancel when we'd planned to get together. But then she admitted something else. "It's hard for me to talk about my cancer now because it's back. I don't want my children to know."

"Maybe this isn't a good time," I said. "It sounds like you need to focus on yourself and your children."

It seemed, however, that she wanted to talk. Sue told me she had wanted to write about her experience but had been too sick to write while she was going through chemotherapy and the stem cell transplant. Now, she was too busy to write.

"Maybe you could write about why so many young women from our mountain area are being diagnosed with breast cancer," she suggested. She knew of a teacher at the preschool, another mother of a child at the elementary school, and two more women in our neighborhood, all who'd been diagnosed. One had already passed away.

Sue thought perhaps it was because of the high radon concentration in our community. "We need to get the radon out of our water and the air because it's not the seventy- and eighty-year-old women who are being diagnosed. It's the thirty- and forty-year-olds, and the ones with babies. We need to get the word out to doctors, too. They're unaware that breast cancer is occurring in so many young women."

Although there was a hint of ire in Sue's voice, she came across more concerned than angry. Soon, she was telling me her story.

"No one would believe me in 1995 when I kept saying there was something wrong with my breast," she said. "It was swollen and painful. I was thirty-five years old and pregnant with my daughter Kayla. The obstetrician said, 'You're pregnant. It's just normal breast changes.' He told me not to worry."

Sue kept complaining about her breast throughout her pregnancy. "I wanted to believe my doctor was right, that it was just from the pregnancy, but, really, I knew something was *not* right."

After her daughter was born, the problems continued as she struggled to breastfeed her. Although they had success on one side, when the baby tried to nurse on the swollen breast, it was too hard. "It was painful, and there was no milk flowing." The problem continued until, finally, Sue begged her doctor at the hospital to check it out. "It's just a blocked duct," he said. "Put hot packs on it." Frustrated, Sue tried refusing to leave the hospital until someone else checked it but was informed that the insurance would not pay for any extra time in the hospital.

"I tried to believe that it was only blocked milk ducts," Sue said, "but by October I was back at the doctor's office with the same complaint. They said that my skin did look strange and agreed there was no milk production, so I was referred to a radiologist for an ultrasound. The radiologist agreed that it looked odd but couldn't see any obvious tumor. We know now that it was because the whole breast was already involved. At the time he thought the reason it looked odd was because I was nursing. I was told to get a mammogram when I finished nursing. When I asked if I should stop nursing, he said, 'There's no hurry.'

"By February of '96 my arm was going numb. I decided then to go to another doctor, and I chose a cancer surgeon. Before I saw the surgeon I told his nurse that I'd had this problem for a year and a half. When the doctor saw me, he said, 'It doesn't look normal, but I can't see a tumor.' He admitted he wasn't used to looking at nursing breasts. Adamantly, I said, 'I need someone who *is* familiar with nursing breasts.'

"His nurse knew right away something was wrong when she saw my breast. She saw the dimpling in my skin and declared, 'You have Peau d'Orange.'"

Peau d'Orange was a bad sign. It meant a locally advanced cancer. With spread to the skin, there was a high probability that microscopic cancer cells had already scattered elsewhere in her body. It was obvious this was a serious case.

The surgeon sent Sue for a needle biopsy right away. The biopsy confirmed an aggressive ductal carcinoma had infiltrated into her skin. Sue's breast cancer was staged at IIIB. All breast cancers that have spread to the skin or chest wall are automatically given this status. The only stage higher, stage IV, is when there is confirmed metastasis to other organs.

They didn't yet know the size or extent of Sue's tumor; however, it was clear that a hard line attack of high-dose chemotherapy followed by a stem cell transplant was imminent. At that time only the most serious and difficult-to-treat cases, such as inflammatory breast cancer and those with ten or more positive nodes, were referred by doctors for stem cell or bone marrow transplants. Insurance companies were *only* considering these cases since the treatment was still considered experimental.

"I needed a mastectomy, too, and since the tumor was so large, I would have to go on chemotherapy first, to shrink the tumor," Sue said. "I was anxious to start the chemotherapy. I really wanted to fight it, and I was happy to finally be doing something about the tumor."

While nursing a one-year-old, mothering a four-year-old, and working full-time an hour from home, Sue began a regimen of eight cycles of CAF—Cytoxan, Adriamycin, and 5-fluorouracil.

"Kayla was nine months old, and I had to stop nursing her cold turkey when I started on the drugs," Sue said. "The weaning was harder on me than for her. I didn't want to break that bond. Fortunately, Kayla readily adapted to the bottle." Initially, Sue started taking her treatments on Thursdays, so she could be back to work on Mondays. Soon, however, she found that the chemotherapy made her nauseated and tired. She was achy and unable to take care of the children on the weekends. "For my kids it was more important that I felt better on the weekends, so I switched my chemotherapy treatments to Mondays."

At work, where she ran computer programs for engineers, she took Ibuprofen when she felt bad. "I lived off of Ibuprofen during that time, and they allowed me some leeway. They gave me the 'busy work,' like filling out forms, where I didn't have to think too much. And later, when I lost my hair, they let me work from home. But even though my hair fell out, I felt like the drugs weren't strong enough. I wanted something more."

Sue would get more. In May she underwent a mastectomy but not yet the reconstruction. "Reconstruction wasn't recommended for me at the time of my mastectomy," she said. "I don't think anyone believed I was going to make it, because when I asked about reconstruction, my oncologist said, 'Let's get through all of your treatment first.' I guess he wanted me to focus on getting well."

At the time of the mastectomy, her surgeon went ahead and removed lymph nodes for dissection as well, which revealed what they had all feared. There was extensive involvement. More than thirteen nodes were positive for the cancer.

Sue would have two months to recover; then, she would start the very high-dose treatment and stem cell transplant. For breast cancer, only the stem cells needed to be harvested and then reinfused. The bone marrow was only necessary in treatment of leukemia. For a patient to be eligible for a stem cell transplant, she must have a severely poor prognosis yet be healthy enough to withstand the effects of the high-dose chemotherapy. Sue met this criteria, and further she understood that the procedure itself could be life threatening. Infection and bleeding were possible complications. She was also aware that menopause, lung problems, or even leukemia were potential side effects of the treatment, and that long-term effects were unknown.

Fortunately for Sue, there was no wait for a bed on the Bone Marrow Transplant Unit, only a wait for approval from her insurance company. The approval came in July, and so did her transplant.

"By then I'd quit my job because my company relocated to Houston. I needed to stay here for treatment, so I accepted their offer of one-year severance pay, and I left."

For three weeks during the month of July, Sue was confined to a sterile room on the Bone Marrow Transplant unit of the University Hospital in Denver. She explained what was required in preparation for the transplant. "I had to get injections of a synthetic growth factor to stimulate my bone marrow to produce more white cells. Then I had a central venous catheter inserted into my chest. When I had enough healthy stem cells releasing from my bone marrow, I went back to the hospital every day for a week, for apheresis."

Here, her blood was drawn from the catheter in her chest into a machine that separated the stem cells in the blood from the other components. "The apheresis made me shaky," Sue remembered. "They gave me lots of Tums."

Her precious stem cells were then safely frozen, hopefully uncontaminated by any tumor cells. Later, after her high-dose chemotherapy, they would be thawed and reinfused into her. Once back into her blood stream, the stem cells would help regenerate tissue damaged by the high-dose chemotherapy. Like no other cells in the body, the immature stem cells had the ability to metamorphose into any kind of cell.

"Six of us had apheresis together," Sue said. "Another woman was also from Conifer. I met her first at our bone marrow orientation, where they showed us the unit and explained everything to us. I remember a deaf woman in our group, too. I tried to talk to her using the bit of sign language I knew, but it was hard. I felt sorry for her. Another girl got an infection during the apheresis, and she had to quit and go home. She was going to have to start all over after she got better."

After enough of her stem cells had been collected and frozen, Sue was admitted to a private room to begin five days of high-dose chemotherapy. It started with seventy-two hours of cisplatin administered through her central venous catheter along with Cytoxan once a day for three days. Other drugs were to control her nausea, and large volumes of IV fluids protected her kidneys and bladder.

"I brought books, a radio, and a tape player to play my swing music," Sue said. "I found out right away I couldn't concentrate enough to read or watch TV. I played my swing music and listened to the radio under my pillow so I wouldn't bother other people. Then, I just wanted to take showers. The shower was the only thing that felt good. I wanted one two or three times a day. Soon, I was hoarding towels because the cleaning staff kept taking them away. They couldn't speak any English, so I had to figure out ways to keep them from taking my towels. I felt like a kid sneaking around.

"After a couple of days on the high-dose chemo, I started getting weaker. I used a stool to sit on in the shower. Once, I stood up and bumped my head on the soap dish that jutted out from the tiled wall. It hurt, but I didn't want to tell the staff because I thought they'd get mad at me for taking so many showers." Later on, when the sore felt better, I told them about it, and they did get mad. 'You could have gotten an infection,' they said.

"I couldn't sleep much, either, during that time because they were taking my blood several times during the night. Then the fifth and last day of chemotherapy was absolute hell. They warned me it would be but kept saying, 'Don't worry, you'll never remember it.'"

It was called hell day for a reason. After two hours on the drug carmustine, Sue was disoriented, vomiting, and had lost bowel control. "The only thing I remember is hurling all over the poor nurse."

With this brutal onslaught of chemotherapy came the risk of developing infections afterward. The high-dose drugs meant to kill all her cancer cells wiped out her white blood cells, leaving her with no immune system at all to fight infections. Another dangerous potential problem was a drug-induced inflammation of the lungs, called interstitial pneumonitis. This could develop any time, even up to two years after her transplant. Without any blood platelets, Sue was also at risk for bleeding problems. It was a time for extreme caution.

Two days after the day of hell came "Day Zero." It was the day her stem cells were thawed and reinfused into her ravaged body. Reinfusing them took only twenty minutes. After that, they began counting each day forward as "days survived" since her stem cell transplant.

For the next two weeks Sue remained in sterile isolation, recuperating while her immature stem cells proliferated and grew into red and white blood cells and blood clotting platelets. The doctors monitored her white cell count as it began to climb back from zero. When it became high enough to protect her again, Sue could go home.

"After Day Zero, I started playing my music again," Sue remembered. "Swing music had always made me want to dance, but I couldn't dance. I was too weak. I dragged myself out of the bed and over to the recliner chair. I could only dance with my fingers on the arm of the chair."

Several more days passed until she began feeling stronger. "I could tell when I was getting stronger because one morning, as I played my swing music, I began to dance around the room. I was thrilled because I thought I was doing well, and then Dr. Jones caught me dancing. 'You can't do that,' he said. 'You could fall.'

"Another day there was a tornado warning, and all of the patients had to be moved from our isolation rooms out into the hallway. Up until that time we'd only seen people in masks and gloves, and now we were seeing each other for the first time since the apheresis stage. Many of us were losing hair. I was losing mine for the second time."

The day finally came for Sue to go home. "I was so happy to be with my kids and husband again, to begin *out-patient* daily monitoring. They said I was a poster girl for stem cell transplants," she bragged, "because after I got the drug to stimulate my white blood cell production [Neupogen], my count came up quickly. I was finished with the out-patient program in less than two weeks." The central venous catheter in her chest came out then, too.

Sue was pleased she'd done well. One woman in her group didn't improve while they were there. "I don't know what hap-

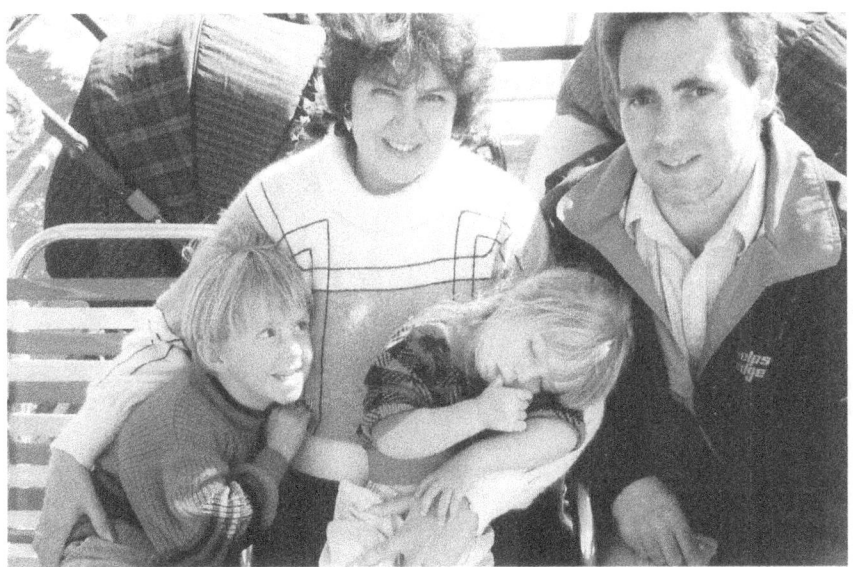

Sue and Mark Niksic, with their children, Shane and Kayla.

pened to her," Sue said. "She and I didn't talk to each other much, and the other woman from Conifer didn't make it. She died soon after her transplant, with a one-year-old baby at home."

Sue's story gave me goose bumps. It was a sobering thought that some had felt themselves forced to choose the high-dose chemotherapy and stem cell transplant—a drastic measure to stay alive for their children's sake—and then lost.

By this time I'd met many breast cancer survivors and heard their stories. Although many of us were doing well after our treatment, as Sue and I would continue our conversations over the telephone, I found out that this disease can be mean and unpredictable. Together, we sisters had to be watchful, and we had to fight.

CHAPTER 30

Waiting and Watching the CEA

Sue survived her stem cell transplant in 1996 and soon thereafter her hair started to grow back. "It came in longer and thicker than it had ever been before," she told me over the phone one day. In spite of the fact that her memory was not quite the same as it had been before chemotherapy, she was enjoying her family and getting on with her life. She got a new job and, even though doctors were monitoring her monthly, she tried to put the breast cancer out of her mind.

"I wore a prosthesis to work, and everything was fine in the daytime, but every night when I took a shower, the mastectomy scar was a reminder," Sue said. "I didn't like it. For three years after the mastectomy, I never changed my mind about wanting reconstruction of my breast. I wasn't happy with only one breast, and my husband and I thought it was a ticking time bomb anyway, so I decided to have a prophylactic mastectomy and an immediate double reconstruction. Since I was healthy, my doctors saw no problem with my decision, so in February of 1999 I went ahead with it."

A plastic surgeon had recommended a double free flap from her abdomen. "I had the Cadillac of surgeries," she bragged. "Fifteen hours." In the operation the surgeon removed two breast-sized sections of tissue from her abdomen and then relocated them under the skin in her chest where her natural breasts had been. Using a microscope to see the tiny blood vessels, he sewed the severed veins and arteries to existing vessels in her armpits, giving a blood supply to the newly transplanted tissues.

Although the results of her reconstruction would eventually make Sue very happy, they would not come easily. Recurrent infections throughout the year required her to go back for more surgeries in February, August, and again in November. It would be a full year until her reconstruction healed. "I'm glad I did it," Sue said. "Though I have no sensation in them, they're real to me, and I think it's important to have breasts."

After the reconstruction came follow-up examinations every six months and blood tests every three months to check her tumor markers. And as with most other people who have had cancer and have finished treatment, she had to learn how to live with the fear of whether it would return. Over time, as her tumor markers remained steady, Sue saw her fear diminish. For twenty-six months there were no signs of recurrence.

"Then in April of 2001 I noticed a strange exhaustion that would come over me suddenly in the evenings," she said. "It was so intense I couldn't even move." Blood tests revealed an elevated CEA. "We knew my cancer was back."

A full-body CT scan located a spot in her liver. "The procedure for the biopsy on my liver was awful," she said. "The doctor wanted me awake so I could breathe in and out at the right times while he probed into my liver during the scan. Supposedly, everything was numb, but it hurt real bad." The biopsy results were negative for cancer. "The doctor didn't trust those results, though, so I had to go through the whole procedure again."

Sue felt lucky to have been sedated the second time. It made the procedure easier, but this time the results came back positive. With tumors in her liver, the cancer was now metastatic. "I have a bunch of tumors in my liver," Sue said. "I'm on hormones now, Arimidex."

Sue's tumor markers remained steady on the Arimidex. "Besides feeling tired and having some pressure in my belly, I'm doing okay," she said.

Sue was dogmatic as to the reason so many women have breast cancer. "We took birth control pills, which are hormones, and then we wanted to have babies, so we took more hormones to get pregnant. We overloaded our bodies with the hormones that feed cancer."

As we were talking, Sue suddenly broke from our telephone conversation to tend to her cooking. "My dinner's boiling over," she said. We'd been on the phone so long, my dinner was overcooking, too, in the oven.

When she returned to the phone, she apologized. "Sorry, I get scatterbrained sometimes. I used to have a good memory, but now I have nothing. Coping with cancer was almost easier when I was on the chemotherapy, because I felt like I was doing something."

Although her cancer was stabilized on Arimidex, she was like all Americans after September 11th—getting on with life while remaining vigilant. Sue knew that for the rest of her life she would always be waiting and watching the CEA.

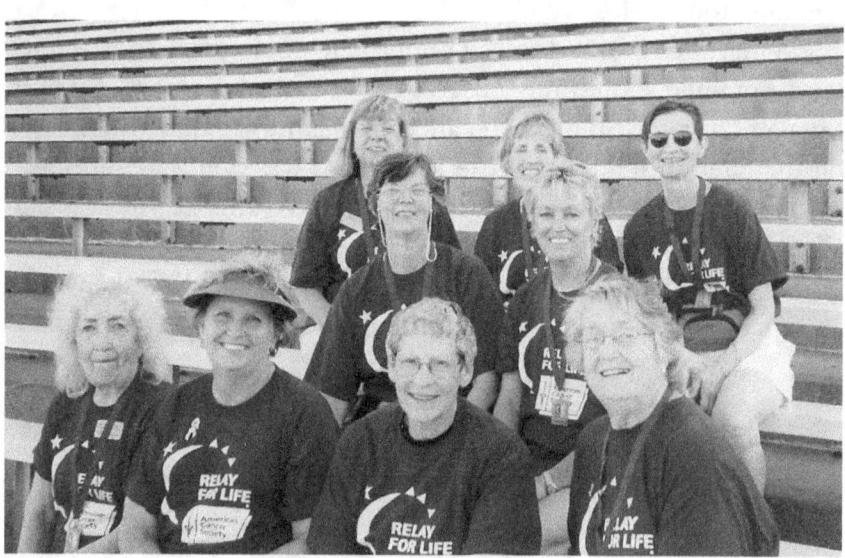

The Association of Breast Cancer Survivor's Relay For Life Team, June 2003. *Top row:* Joyce Coville, Anne Baird, Penny Cooper. *Second row:* Sandy Weaver, Ruth McMahon. *Bottom row:* Marion Patton, RoseMary Ashford, Harriette Grober, Pat Grahn.

CHAPTER 31

A Matter of Hope

Unlike Sue, with a cure rate of close to one hundred percent for my in situ cancer, I didn't spend much time worrying about my cancer coming back. Although I know that having been diagnosed with cancer twice, I am at high risk for developing a new cancer, I don't dwell on it. Still, the words of Dr. Christine Rogness, a general surgeon, have stayed with me since I heard her speak on a panel at my first Day of Caring: "We love all of our patients, but we get especially close to our breast cancer patients," she said. "We follow them for a long time because it's not a matter of *if* their cancer comes back; it's a matter of *when*."

It is a fact we live with. Many people believe we need a positive attitude to yield a positive outcome with cancer. I hear them remark that their friend or relative "has such a positive attitude." I wonder—what choice do we have? Most of us want to live. Survival is a natural instinct, so we say, "I'm going to beat this."

We do feel scared, angry, and depressed, fatigued and out of control, trying to hang on to life when it's threatened to be taken too soon. But living like that becomes too cumbersome. It's easier to focus on the moment. In the moment you see more clearly how green a single blade of grass is and how sweet a rose and how dear a friend. And that is where we get our positive attitude. It is the gift we get from cancer.

A positive attitude doesn't guarantee survival. I know of people who did all of the right things, including eating right, were vegetarians, went to church, remained positive, and were generally "good" people, yet succumbed nevertheless. People say they "lost the battle."

I never felt like I was battling anything. I never felt sick. I would have been incensed if people said I was "battling" cancer. Besides a difficult, body-altering surgery, for me there was never really a fight. At first, I didn't like being thrown into the category of "breast cancer survivor." After I came out of the hospital, I was still wavering in denial that I was one. I said to my brother, "Nobody has ever called me a 'melanoma survivor'; why should I be called a 'breast cancer survivor'?" He just looked at me blankly. He had no answer.

But Harriette has said it has felt like a battle for her. She said, "When I have a setback, I say 'I've got to win this,' and then I fight till I come to a plateau again."

My grandmother did battle breast cancer, and my mother battled against Parkinson's disease. People battle against depression, schizophrenia, and diabetes, too. Each of us has our challenges. Although many people will say they're not glad they have cancer, they feel their lives have been enriched by it.

Before breast cancer, Kim, Pat, Harriette, Sue, and I were ordinary Colorado residents, with nothing else in common. Then we each faced this demon that behaves and manifests itself in different ways. Our breast cancers are different, as are our lifestyles and our ages, but we each experience the same thoughts about our mortality and the same grief, anger, denial, bargaining, depression, and acceptance. And we each receive and embrace the gifts that cancer gives us: an added richness to our lives of new friends and new starts and the ability to appreciate each new day and to see things in a new light. We seek to live out each day to the fullest, never again taking the future for granted but looking forward with optimism and hope.

As time passes there are plenty of days when I forget I ever had breast cancer. I catch myself slipping back into old habits—getting irritated over small things that seem important, like scratches on the car, stains on the carpet, or wasting time in traffic or in lines at the pharmacy. I start worrying too much about tomorrow instead of enjoying today. The only things we have are today and our hope for tomorrow.

From cancer I've learned not to put off till tomorrow what I can do today, and so I have written this book. Joyce Coville was instrumental in helping me adopt this attitude. Her positive influence pushed me forward the first day, when as President of the Association of Breast Cancer Survivors, she welcomed me into the group. Having survived breast cancer since 1987, Joyce exudes an upbeat and positive attitude about life after breast cancer. "We certainly want to support you in writing that book," she'd said when I told her what I had in mind.

At a subsequent meeting I heard Joyce offer encouragement to another tearful, two-month post-op survivor. "It gets better," Joyce said, putting her arm around the woman. Joyce opened my eyes and heart to the idea that life after breast cancer can be better than life before breast cancer. Now, when I see thousands flock to the Race for the Cure, the Relay for Life, and the Avon 3-Day Walks, I see a sea of hope.

But in our hope, even Joyce Coville, our fearless leader, gets down sometimes. During our telephone conversation one day in April 2003, she sounded distraught. "I'm worried about Harriette," she told me. "I heard she's had progression." Joyce's sister was also suffering from breast cancer. "It's in my sister's lungs," Joyce said. Her voice was different from her usual cheerful tone. "I don't know what to do for Harriette or for my sister. I went to my sister's home in Texas to be with her, and I ended up ill with chest pains and diarrhea. I don't think I was of any help to her." Joyce felt it was her own anxiety that had caused her illness. "It's really different when it's one of your own family members," she said. "I think I can deal with it easier when it's me than I can when it's my sister."

I reminded Joyce she did do something for her sister. "You went there to be with her, and she knows that." I suspected that Joyce had given much to others over the years, too.

As I write this, three years have passed since my diagnosis, and I can say I've changed. I'm proud to be a breast cancer survivor. I'm proud to be one of the sisters. I focus my energy on learning and writing, and I'm still reading all I can about breast cancer. I've learned that in the thirty years since my grandmother's diagnosis, treatments have improved but not changed significantly. The same chain of events that happened to Grandma are not unheard of today. The biggest difference is that our awareness and understanding of this disease have greatly increased.

Historically, society blamed this disease on the woman herself for her transgressions or her weak emotional state. And early treatment consisted of mere blood letting or topical pastes made of arsenic and zinc chloride. When these and other more barbaric treatments failed, the woman faced her hideous tumors alone while they spread furiously over and throughout her body. The woman was left to suffer a sure and painful death.

With modern treatments, there's no reason for any woman ever to have to see cancer manifest itself in an ugly black rage across her body. Today we strive for earlier detection in women by encouraging routine mammograms, and with improved technology we're achieving this objective. We're advocating for less mutilating treatments for breast cancer, more efficient cures, and the provision of healthcare for all women. But most importantly we are fervently asking "Why?" Why are women getting breast cancer? When we can answer this question, we will know how to prevent it from occurring in the first place. Until we know the answer, it's difficult to pinpoint preventions. Yet, we're doing what we believe we must with the information we have.

Fifty-nine medicines are currently in various stages of testing for breast cancer by pharmaceutical researchers. There is certainly reason for hope in the eradication of breast cancer, perhaps even in my lifetime. It's this matter of hope that keeps pushing Joyce, Harriette, Kim, Pat, Sue, me, and the sisterhood forward.

CHAPTER 32

Burning Questions

―――◆―――

Tulips usually mean the arrival of spring. At our altitude on Conifer Mountain, we don't have any tulips growing to tell us that. It's usually the rain and the sound of water rushing down the stream lining our property and, of course, the longer days with daylight savings time. After the bone-dry winter of 2002, however, there was no loud rush of water in our stream. There was only more sunlight. But even without the rushing stream or the tulips, for me spring always means new starts, celebrations, and the anticipation of resolving answers to questions.

In May that year we proudly celebrated Heather's graduation from Colorado State University in Fort Collins. To mark her start into the adult world, we had a party at the house she shared with her roommates. We took pictures in the yard, in front of the blooming lilacs, and then the party guests began asking the question of our new graduate, "Now what are you going to do?" She didn't know. Maybe she would get a job in her field of social work, or she would go back to teaching gymnastics or apply to graduate school. Or maybe she would get her ailing tonsils removed first.

The same weekend of Heather's graduation I attended the Day of Caring for breast cancer survivors. Although I was hoping to see Kim and Harriette there, I hadn't expected to meet up with Kim in the parking lot. We pulled into our spaces nose to nose at the same time. We were both arriving a bit late, and we'd missed the

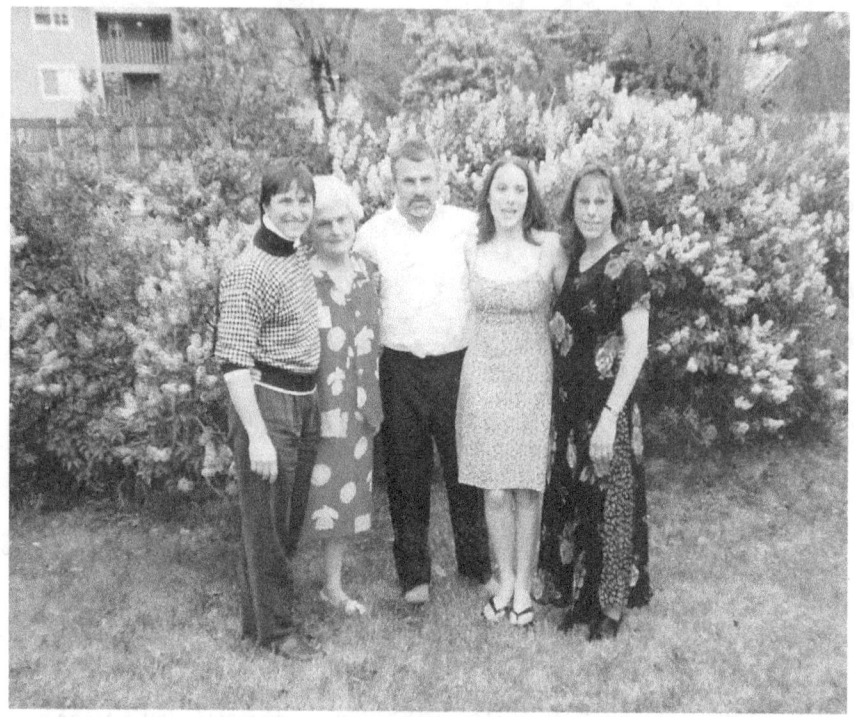

Heather's graduation from Colorado State University, 2002.

welcoming session, but at least she was in time to hook up with her friend, Sarah McClintock, in the mezzanine.

As always, I was interested in meeting other survivors, especially Sarah, whom I'd heard so much about from Kim. It had saddened and stilled my heart when I came to know of the drastic situation she'd faced and what she'd been through. At the same time it filled me with hope. Like Kim, Sarah had also been diagnosed at age twenty-eight, and they both had had the same surgeon. In fact, it was their surgeon who urged Kim to make the call that brought the two of them together. They became friends instantly while Sarah was on an urgent mission to preserve her chance of having children before starting chemotherapy.

Since it was possible that the toxic drugs could render her infertile, Sarah had availed herself of the only medical options she had, even knowing they were still experimental: drugs to protect her ovaries and freezing of her embryos. Because it's not known whether human eggs are as viable after the thaw, as embryos are, Sarah and her husband had chosen to take the first step of in vitro fertilization, and then had the embryos frozen, in case they would need them later.

Kim had been a huge moral support to Sarah during the month when she and her husband underwent the $12,000 process, which according to Sarah, "proceeded so quickly, we had little time to mull over choices." Without delay they had had to research the subject and make difficult decisions. Sarah had taken hormone injections to hyperstimulate her ovaries to produce eggs. Days later, she underwent general anesthesia for the surgery to harvest as many of her eggs as possible. The eggs were then fertilized in the laboratory by her husband's sperm, and the embryos frozen.

For Sarah and her husband the process netted only three embryos. The precious three would be all they would have because the oncologist had approved only one round of extraction of eggs before starting her chemotherapy. Her cancer was hormone responsive, and it wasn't known whether the hormone injections taken during the in-vitro process were also feeding her tumor. Her chemotherapy needed to start as soon as possible.

From the hormones and chemotherapy came symptoms of medically induced menopause. When Sarah experienced hot flashes and insomnia, Kim had been there to lend emotional support, having been down that road herself.

Today, with all her treatment behind her, Sarah was with Kim, attending her first Day of Caring. Very petite, in a leopard print skirt, she looked to me like a model with her big round eyes and adorably short, wet-look haircut—which, I quickly realized, wasn't a haircut at all. It was the inch-long outgrowth following her final chemotherapy treatment.

Since the first track of seminars had already started, I suggested we hurry. In a flash we scanned the program book for the selection of choices. We each picked the same one: "Breast Cancer News and New Treatments—What's Hot and What's Not" and scurried down the hall to locate the room. Fortunately, the meeting hadn't started yet. People were still visiting in small clusters. I noticed Dr.

McAleese, who was to be on one of the panels, heading over to greet us. At the same time I spotted Harriette talking to some other women we knew from the American Cancer Society. There was still time to say hello to her.

"I'm not doing well," Harriette told me. The corners of her mouth turned down. She seemed thinner although I thought she looked beautiful in an elegant blue-gray pantsuit. Her cheeks were flushed. "The Arimidex has stopped working," she said. She knew because the pain in her hip was back. "I started Taxotere yesterday."

I knew she hadn't wanted to do that. I hugged her and promised we'd get together in a few days.

I kept thinking about Harriette while our first speaker talked about a new method of radiation called brachytherapy, where a radioactive seed is implanted into the tumor site. The seed releases a succinct dose to a localized area in just five days. Brachytherapy was being tested to see whether it's more effective than traditional radiation. I guessed that brachytherapy was a good thing, yet the word itself sounded creepy to me. I hoped I'd never need it.

In his lecture the speaker emphasized something I thought we all needed to hear because, often, I'd hear a woman wondering why her friend got a treatment different from her own. "Breast cancer is not just one disease for which clinicians can treat everyone the same," he said. In his last remark he said that studies had shown intensive surveillance by routine laboratory tests and scans to detect recurrences had not made any difference in survival rates over regular surveillance by annual examinations and mammography. It reminded me that I hadn't had any of the follow-up blood tests or chest X-rays that had been recommended for me.

We heard next on "The Latest in Hormonal Therapies" from an oncology expert who, I'd read, carried a case load of more than one thousand patients. He was vivacious and charismatic, talking with his hands while he enlightened us about the benefits of first-line drugs such as tamoxifen and Arimidex. First-line drugs are those prescribed first to inhibit the cancer. If there is a relapse or progression of the cancer on one of the first-line drugs, you switch to another drug. There are others that can be used in hormone therapy as second, third, or fourth lines, such as Faslodex, Megace, Premarin, Halotestin, and Exemestane. The newest drug, Faslodex, he said completely inhibits estrogen receptors. These drugs were his main lines of defense, and his protocol was to prescribe them consecutively. "Halotestine, a male hormone, makes you feel *strong*," he said, emphasizing the word by drawing it out. "You go to work, and you don't take crap from anyone. And none of my patients has had to shave yet."

He prescribed Faslodex as his third line of defense. "We don't use it up front," he said. In his opinion it was a great drug for metastatic breast cancer. "I tend to use hormones, hormones, and hormones. Then if there's a recurrence, we can move on to chemotherapy. Women don't like to get that shot in the butt," he said, "and fortunately for them, I have many options up my sleeve. Even if the tumor markers are going up, I treat the patient, not the numbers. A few little spots on your bones are not going to kill you. I wait for the cancer to force me to change my therapy."

Next to me, Kim raised her hand. She asked, "What if your tumor is ER negative and you have a recurrence?" From his convoluted answer, it seemed to me that there was little recourse, since ER negative tumors didn't respond to hormones. The only choice would be to go to a second-line chemotherapy. The answer didn't fill me with optimism. I guessed it hadn't felt satisfactory to Kim either because later she asked me whether I thought he had answered her question.

"It didn't seem like it," I said. We left with the question still gnawing at us. Her tumor had been ER negative.

When the first Day of Caring was held twenty-one years ago, there were thirty-five attendees. This year, there were a thousand of us. At noon we gathered around one hundred tables, set below a stage, for the annual luncheon and fashion show. I sat with Harriette and Lois Hjelmstad, whose quilt had hung with Harriette's at the *common threads* exhibit. I felt honored to be among these women, who had done so much for the cause. Like Harriette, Lois was well known in the breast cancer community as an outspoken advocate. As an author, she spoke on breast cancer issues throughout the United States and England.

Sue Miller, the Day of Caring founder and thirty-year breast cancer survivor, welcomed us. White-haired now, she stood before us, tall and stunningly beautiful in a bright red jacket. We honored her with a full applause for her recent induction into the Colorado Women's Hall of Fame. Every year at the Day of Caring an award is given in Sue Miller's name to honor individuals in the community who have done exemplary work in the fight against breast cancer. This year, Harriette Grober was called to accept the award.

Harriette stood radiantly at the microphone. "I'm honored to accept this award on behalf of fourteen of us from the Colorado Breast Cancer Coalition who have produced the Colorado Breast Cancer Resources Directory," she said. In a labor-intensive endeavor, her group, including Cyndi Grober, had placed numerous calls to keep the directory updated since its inception in 1995, when it consisted of only ten pages. Now the directory was thirty-five pages, and twelve thousand copies had been printed, in Spanish as well as English. It listed nearly every resource in Colorado related to breast cancer, complete with where to go for medical information, where to find support services, and suggested reading. With the effort of people like these, the breast cancer community had come a long way since Grandma Shaver's time.

When the yearly fashion show began, I saw that Aimee Sporer was moderating again, but this time she had a partner—Charlie Blosten, who was himself a breast cancer survivor. I remembered him as one of the models from last year. All of the models were breast cancer survivors from our local community.

Charlie introduced the first model. There were a dozen models, including a couple of men. Unlike the year before, I was able to enjoy this fashion show. Where I'd felt it was an exploitation of their tragedies then, I was truly celebrating these survivors. I understood the positive side of breast cancer now—friendship, living with purpose, and love. I could be more upbeat.

At the end, all of the models convened for a final promenade down the runway, dancing to Kool and the Gang's "Celebration." Everyone joined in clapping, and I sang along. At the close, when people were dispersing, I rushed to the stage to get Charlie's attention. "I'm writing about breast cancer," I told him after I'd introduced myself. "Would you be interested in talking to me about it, as a male survivor?" With all the noise, he had to bend down so he could hear me better. "Yes, sure," he said and handed me a business card, which indicated he worked for the City of Littleton.

"My husband's aunt used to work there," I said. "Maybe you know her." Coincidentally, he did know her. "She had breast cancer, too," I said, realizing the second coincidence, "twenty years ago." I told Charlie I would call him as I ran off to catch the last session of the afternoon.

After a lively luncheon, it was a somber afternoon when members of the audience posed questions to a panel of medical experts. A few women with no hair were scattered among us. One of them wanted to know if everyone is reconstructable and if scar tissue is a problem in delayed reconstruction. Another woman complained of uncomfortable side effects from both tamoxifen and Arimidex. "What else can I take?" she asked.

Others asked questions like: Why can't lobular cancer be diagnosed by mammography? How accurate is a sentinel node biopsy for multi-focal disease? What is ductal lavage? What about hyperbaric therapy? These were burning questions. We'd brought them to the Day of Caring, hoping to leave with answers.

CHAPTER 33

Scared

"No lifeguard on duty"
it is difficult when one is drowning
to wave to the people on shore
one wants to be friendly, of course,
but perhaps it is more important to keep swimming
   Lois Tschetter Hjelmstad, excerpt from *Fine Black Lines*

On Monday I was tooling down the highway when my phone rang. It was Harriette calling from the hotel where her family was staying. "You agreed to meet me for breakfast at my place," she reminded me. "I'm calling to schedule the day."

Two days later I was knocking on her hotel room door at ten minutes to eight in the morning. It surprised me when her two little dogs answered with their barking. I'd never heard barking dogs in a hotel before, and when no one came to the door, I winced at their continuing noise. I didn't want to be the cause of the bother to sleeping neighbors. A couple of minutes later, I was relieved when I saw Harriette coming down the hall. In a tank top and gym shorts, her skin shone moist from perspiration. It was obvious she'd been in the workout room.

"You're early," she said. "I should have known; you're always early. Stanley's still asleep."

"He's not now," I said, referring to the barking.

Inside their suite, Harriette handed me the report of her recent bone scan and told me to read it while she went to shower.

Snow, her white cock-a-poo, and Rascal, the scraggly seven-pound affenpinscher, hadn't yet calmed down. Snow continued her barking and tried to jump in my lap when I sat down. She quieted only when I pet her, so I rubbed her tummy her as I read.

The report was not good news, and I was worried. It said: "Extensive osseous metastatic disease is present as noted. The disease has progressed since last exam. Now, new and larger lesions in skull, thoracic, lumbar spine, pelvis, ribs, and progression in left proximal femur with possible impending fracture."

After her shower, we walked together with Stanley to the common area of the hotel for breakfast. "I'm scared," Harriette admitted when we sat down at the table. "The medicine, Taxotere, makes my stomach distend, and it hurts."

The steroids, Decadron, given with Taxotere to prevent swelling in the legs, were making her gain weight. The doctor had told Harriette she wanted her to stay on Taxotere for six months. She said the chemotherapy would probably only work for eight to ten months. Harriette told me she didn't want to stay on the IV chemotherapy.

"What do you want to do?" I asked.

"I'd rather go back on hormones," she said. "I want Faslodex, but I don't know what to do. Jeff and I are supposed to go on a seventy-five-mile bike ride this Sunday."

There were so many roads to choose, and life depended on which one you chose, she thought. "Garfield had me on 5fU, the oldest, cheapest, most benign therapy. He just left it alone, and it worked for nine and a half years. Some of those years were hell because of conflicts in the family, and six years ago I wouldn't have cared if I had died, but I lived. He let me live in denial. Then I became so confident I was going to live, I cashed out all my life insurance policies. They were only good until age seventy anyway, and I thought, surely, I would live to seventy."

Harriette's new oncologist, Dr. Hinshaw, was always doing scans and blood work and was quick to make changes. She didn't let Harriette live in denial. Harriette wasn't so sure this way was better. She asked Dr. Hinshaw whether she should start looking for alternative care for Cyndi.

"Not yet," she answered.

Harriette knew Cyndi was scared too. "I just want to live," Harriette continued. "I want to be here for Cyndi, and I want to ride my bike. But sooner or later all cells have the ability to get around what it is that's trying to stop them."

Her tumors had been dumb for a long time. Now they were getting smart again. She was considering whether to undergo more radiation, wondering whether it would do her more harm than good. "My radiologist hasn't seen anyone like me before," she said. "I'm always off their bell curve."

She knew her doctors had her best interests at heart. Harriette herself was becoming more interested in her quality of life at this point. She wanted to ride her new bike. She'd ridden it only four times. The last time was two days ago, when she and Jeff had taken an evening ride from Confluence Park to Washington Park, where the two of them stopped to rest on a bench. They'd had one of their philosophical talks.

"Jeff thinks it's good that I'm spending time having lunch with friends. He knows that camaraderie is important to me. I love being around people, but when I have a scare like this, sometimes I pull away and stop talking to people."

After their ride to the park, Jeff and Harriette made a customary stop for ice cream at the Bonnie Brae parlor, where a red-and-white-striped awning announces, "Yes! We make it here!" "There are always lines of people there," Harriette said. "We ordered our usual—one waffle cone with coffee and mint-chocolate-chip ice cream, with nuts. We never get one each," she laughed. Outside, they sat on the wrought-iron bench to savor their shared ice cream cone amidst red potted geraniums.

Before she left Stanley and me at the breakfast table to go answer a page, Harriette said the only way she would stay on the chemotherapy was if the cancer was in her lungs. She knew there were many small spots there, but she would see for sure when she got the results of her lung scan the next day.

Alone, Stanley and I looked at each other. We'd never even had a conversation before. In his face I saw a strong resemblance to Cyndi. As much as I cared for Harriette and what she was going through, my heart ached for him, too. So often we forget how cancer in one family member affects the others. We don't stop to think what they're going through. "So, how have you been doing through all of this?" I asked.

He shook his head, and his lips curled down at the corners. I couldn't tell whether he always did that or was trying not to cry. "It's been tough," he said. "*Really* tough. I'm worried now. They're not sure if the chemo will work."

"I bet you've been worried many times."

"Yes, but there were always other drugs to try. Now there aren't. We will have been married forty years in November." I knew they were planning to go to Washington, D.C., in the fall to celebrate their anniversary. Stanley had never been there before.

Harriette returned and picked up the conversation where she'd left off. "I'm torn," she said. "I'll do whatever I have to, to live. I just don't want to use dynamite if a BB gun will work. I'd hate for them to say later, 'Oh, if she only could have hung on one more year, now we have this *great* drug.'"

The next day Harriette called me with her lung scan results. "The scan is the same," she says. "And Dr. Hinshaw went along with my request for Faslodex. I'll be the first person on Coumadin to get it."

Because Faslodex was given by injection, for someone on blood thinning medication there was a greater risk of severe bruising or bleeding at the injection site. Harriette was willing to take the risk and try it. "Because nothing else is working," she said. She would get Faslodex with Taxotere for three months and then totally drop the chemo. "I like her," Harriette added. "She cares about me, and she's an excellent doctor."

CHAPTER 34

The Power of the Mind

It was the end of May, and still it hadn't rained. A thick smoky haze hung in the air. The smoke was from the Schoonover fire, near the town of Deckers, which had been burning for four days and had charred four thousand acres. This fire, sparked by lightning, was the third in a month within a twenty-mile radius of our house. From my home I drove through the smoke, still carrying my most important treasures in the car since the last fire, less than three weeks ago.

The day that fire started I was driving west toward the mountains when I saw the pink-and-orange cloud of smoke, billowing from one of the peaks off in the distance. The smoke appeared to be coming right from the direction of my home. I promptly called Jim on my cell phone. "Is there a fire up there?" He said he didn't think so. He'd been working in the basement, but three minutes later he called me back, yelling into the phone. "It's two miles from here! Get home!"

They were calling it the Black Mountain Fire. For the rest of the afternoon we watched the smoke billow over the mountain behind us and kept abreast of the fire by television while we hosed down dry weeds around the perimeter of the house. We packed the cars with important files, photo albums, and clothing, working as fast as we could. In the late evening the wind turned the Black Mountain Fire toward the west, taking us out of the line of danger. Knowing that helped us fall asleep that night. The next day we learned the fire had been contained. Still, we kept a lookout, wondering when and where the next fire would be.

For the next few days I found myself packing and unpacking belongings, choosing things that were the most important to save from a fire and then deciding which things we could sacrifice. It was hard to focus on anything else. I started feeling guilty for wanting my material things and for not getting anything else done.

Living in a forested area for twenty-three years, where there has always been the possibility of fire, I've learned that the less time you have to get out the easier it is to know which things to take as you leave your house behind. If you have three minutes, you take the photo albums and important files. If you have three hours, you add clothes and things that are dear to you. If you have three days, you practically pack up the whole house.

The drill was another exercise in taking stock of my life—deciding who and what are most important, what is meaningful, and what is not. Maybe it was time to make changes in my life. Like breast cancer, the fire was another wake-up call, a reminder to wade through the unimportant and cherish the remainder.

The smoky haze stretched over the city as far east as the Aurora suburb, where I pulled into the Summerfield Suites parking lot. My eyes and throat were stinging even before I got out of the car. I was meeting Harriet and Stanley for breakfast again. This time, I prepared myself for Snow's and Rascal's barking when I knocked on room number 177. At ten and eleven years old, the little dogs were still pretty spunky.

Harriette greeted me at the door. She and Stanley were both ready to walk me down to the common dining room. They were dressed in all black except for the hot pink top Harriette wore under her pantsuit jacket. "You two are looking spiffy this morning," I commented.

"Because we usher tonight," she said.

From the entrance I caught a shadow of Cyndi in her room, sitting up in bed. There was just enough light on her face to make out the tube that fed oxygen to her lungs. Her empty wheelchair waited near her bed. She wouldn't be able to go outside today. There was too much smoke.

We left her in the suite with Snow and Rascal reminding us that we'd left them behind. Over their barking, Harriette told me she was excited about an "engagement" Cyndi had tonight. She was having a first date with someone she'd met through an online organization for members with disabilities. Stanley remarked that he was anxious to get the dogs back into their own home, where they have "doggie doors." "Even though Snow can pull Cyndi in her wheelchair, it's difficult for her to manage both dogs outside when we aren't here," he said. "She's had both of her shoulders replaced, and they're wearing out."

Over breakfast Harriette and Stanley reminisced about their old dog, Garfield. "He was so smart, he was in a play once, at the temple," Stanley said. "When Cyndi said 'bang, bang,' he would roll over and play dead. People thought it was a crack up."

"Yes, but he got stage fright that day and wouldn't do it in the play," Harriette laughed. "Rascal is so different than him. I've always thought he's autistic because he'll never look you in the eye, and he'd rather be off by himself. But the other day he curled up on the bed with me. I asked Cyndi, 'What's wrong with him?' She said, 'Nothing's wrong with him; he knows there's something wrong with you.'"

Harriette said she felt scared now about her cancer. "I was scared once before, when I was forty-two years old, and then I had the same mental anguish again in '92, when I had my recurrence. I believed nobody survived metastatic disease. But then I put my head in the sand for ten years. I've got my head out of the sand now, and I feel out of control."

She had seen her good friend Judy recently when they had lunch together. Times before, when Harriette was first diagnosed and then again when she found her recurrence, Judy had said, "You'll be okay." She'd had a good feeling about it. Now when Harriette asked her, "Do you have a good feeling now?" she answered, "You've had eighteen years."

"Those eighteen years went by in a flash," Harriette lamented. Listening to her made me think about my Dad. He died when he stopped setting goals in his life. After we buried Mom's ashes in the church playground we had built and dedicated to her, Dad had accomplished his last goal. He passed away not too long after that.

"I think people live as long as they still have goals," I said.

"Good, because Jeff and I are planning a trip to New Zealand in January," she said. "We went to England even when I was in pain. Jeff had to carry my backpack, but we walked through more museums than healthy people do. When you get sick, the grass always looks greener, the mountains seem brighter, and things even *smell* better."

"Are you planning to bike in New Zealand?"

"Yeah, we might rent some bikes there."

Stanley looked over at his wife. "She finished the seventy-five mile ride last Sunday with Jeff," he said. His face beamed with a wide smile that showed the little spaces between his teeth and a few wrinkles at the corner of his bright eyes.

"Do you ride with her?" I asked.

"Not anymore," he said. "I'm just happy she can still do it, and I'm jealous because I can't." Stanley got too short of breath when he rode. His bike was collecting dust.

Harriette and Jeff's bike-touring group had initiated the seventy-five mile ride at 70th and Broadway, where they headed off toward their final destination in Ft. Lupton. The riders planned to refresh themselves on root-beer floats there, at the A&W stop. While they all started off together, riding around the Riverside golf course, the group soon sped ahead of Harriette and Jeff.

"Our leader had said it would be flat the whole way, but there were rolling hills all around the golf course," Harriette complained. "We had an unrelenting headwind, and my legs felt like rubber." Several times she thought they should stop and turn around as they kept pedaling through the cow country. It looked like the road went on forever. Harriette watched for each road marker, riding past the #2 and then the #4. After two hours of pedaling and increasingly short of breath, Harriette came upon #6. Realizing the A&W was at road marker #12, she wondered whether she was going to make it. "We did the talk test. If you can pedal and talk at the same time, then you know you have enough energy. I couldn't talk. Then I saw #6 ½. I'd never used drafting before, but I let Jeff ride just ahead, where he could draft me. He pulled me up the hills."

Finally, she saw a red-and-white sign in the distance. Huffing and puffing, she called out to Jeff, "Do you think that's the A&W?"

He turned his head, yelling back "Yeah, I think so."

It took them three hours to get there, and then they didn't even indulge in the root beer floats. Jeff drank a root beer without ice cream, and Harriette savored an apple. On the way back, without the same bothersome headwind, the ride to 70th and Broadway took only two hours. "At the end of the ride, we high-fived each other and drove off to get some food."

I shook my head in amazement. "How do you do it?" I asked.

"It's the power of the mind," she said. "It's been the power of the mind all along that has gotten me this far. I learned about the power of the mind from QuaLife, at the Break the Board workshop in 1986. The workshop was one of the most meaningful experiences in my life. That and Spa for the Spirit."

I'd never heard of either of these things. "What is Break the Board?"

"It was in 1986, during the first self-help weekend ever offered by the QuaLife Wellness Community," she said. The weekend was designed to help people with cancer or other illnesses to optimize their physical, emotional, social, and spiritual well-being. She and Cyndi were among the first participants to take advantage of the program, founded by the late Dr. Paul K. Hamilton. He was a well-thought-of Denver oncologist, who believed he could *help people regain a line of balance when the world felt out of control.*

"I always like to feel like I'm in control," Harriette said. "The hardest part of the program for me was when we had to be blindfolded and depend on another person to lead us through an obstacle course filled with stairs and narrow walkways."

During the training two workshop leaders taught them how to center themselves. By centering their energy and their focus, they were told they would discover the amazing power of the mind. They would see it working at the end of the workshop when they were to break through thick boards with the side of their hands.

When it came time for this, the participants donned headbands and each one pulled their energy into focus. To vibrant music and clapping, they took turns finding their "center" to break the board using the power of the mind. "One lady wanted to break the board so badly. She tried many times and always missed. Then Cyndi wanted to try. We were worried because her hands are frail, and we thought she might get hurt. But she broke the board on the first try."

Then it was Harriette's turn. With her strong bones and hands she thought she would break it, too, easily. Gathering her strength, she smashed her hand down on the board held tightly by two others. With a jarring halt and sting to her hand, the board held firm.

"I tried again and missed the second time, too," Harriette said. "My hand was sore, but I thought since I'd just had three hours of training, I ought be able to do it. So, I did my mental exercises again and centered my energy. Then my hand came down and went through the board like it was paper."

Ever since that weekend, Harriette had been attending QuaLife gatherings and events, which, later on, were held at the renovated Hamilton House mansion in the Capital Hill neighborhood of Denver. The QuaLife mansion, which had been Dr. Hamilton's dream, was donated to QuaLife after his death from lung cancer. Though Dr. Hamilton never saw his dream come to fruition, Harriette felt endeared to him because QuaLife had made an important difference in her and her family's quality of life.

I wanted to hear more about QuaLife and Spa for the Spirit, but, as morning had come into bloom, Stanley was up from the table preparing to leave. "Go feed the dogs and walk them," Harriette said to him. "And make it a *good* walk."

Although she seemed strong and healthy to me, after Stanley left, she told me she wasn't doing well. Her eyes looked red and irritated. Because the chemotherapy had lowered her resistance, they were infected. The Taxotere had made her mouth sore, and she was having pain.

"Where are you feeling the pain?" I asked.

She ran her hand up and down her thigh. "It's here in my femur. The cancer is all over me, but I don't feel sick. I'm just having this pain. The cancer in my bones won't kill me, but in my lungs, it might."

Jeff had seen his mother limping for two days after their ride. Worried, he had asked her what was wrong. He thought maybe she'd ridden too much. "No," she'd answered, "it isn't that kind of pain." Cyndi was so petrified about what was going to happen to her mother and to herself that she'd been having trouble sleeping. She was telling her mother, "I fought to be here, so you better stay here, too."

These recent symptoms had given Harriette reason to consider alternative placement for Cyndi again. "There's nothing out there," she told me. "We looked at nursing homes again this weekend."

The last time she'd done this was this past winter, after learning of her latest cancer recurrence. Harriette had gone by herself, driving Cyndi's 1991 Astro van equipped with hand controls. Cyndi used to drive the van, until she could no longer transfer herself into the driver's seat. Now Harriette drove it. After visiting a couple of facilities, Harriette had driven away from the last one screaming, *"No, no, no!"* This weekend, all three of them had gone together—to weigh their options.

"The average age of a nursing home resident is eighty years old," Harriette said, "and two-thirds of them are severely developmentally disabled. One place we saw didn't even have cut sidewalks for wheelchairs. A nursing home's just not the right environment for Cyndi. They don't have staff qualified to take care of her. She needs specialists who know what to do for her. She has an iliostomy and a foley catheter. She's on oxygen, and she takes over one hundred pills a day."

Harriette had to order Cyndi's twenty different medications on time to make sure she didn't run out. Medicaid wouldn't pay for them if they were ordered less than thirty days apart, and not all of the medicines could be ordered at the same time. Sometimes medicines in the delivery were missing. Harriette helped keep Cyndi on schedule with the pills because some she took twice a day and others three or four times a day. The pills had to be taken on time, at 7:00 A.M., noon, three o'clock, dinnertime, and at bedtime. Harriette and Cyndi preferred setting up the pills together, because when they had the nurses do them, things often got mixed up.

"I can't put her in a nursing home," Harriette said. "She's petrified, and she's not sleeping. Even sleeping pills aren't helping her." Harriette concluded that if she passed away, the best thing for Cyndi would be to stay in the house with Stanley and to continue to depend on home healthcare, as bad as it often was. "It will be stated in my will that she will have the right to stay in the house as long as she wishes. Or, when I go, I'll just take her with me."

I didn't know what to say to Harriette. Tears were filling my eyes, and I had sudden chills.

CHAPTER 35

Race for the Cure

———

Seeing Charlie Blosten and the other male models at the Day of Caring had impressed upon me that, even though we called it a sisterhood, breast cancer wasn't just a women's disease. Charlie was committed to spreading the word that breast cancer was a men's disease, too. From him I learned how breast cancer affects men.

When they are diagnosed with breast cancer, men have almost the same treatments as women, and they have an equally difficult time—physically and emotionally. It is perhaps even more difficult because of the stigma that this is a female disease. Also, there is less community support for men. Charlie was doing his part to increase awareness about this. When I met with him at his office in the City of Littleton building, I found out what a big part it was.

Charlie, a graying and energetic guy, not much taller than my five foot six, was wrapping up a phone call when I arrived. While I waited, I read the board on the office wall, which listed nearly fifty city projects he was involved with, all in progress. I'd gotten as far as number thirty-eight, the tree replacement program, when he hung up the telephone. For the next hour, in between more phone calls and various other interruptions, Charlie spoke openly to me about his breast cancer.

"I first noticed my lump in January of 1997, on my fiftieth birthday," he said, patting his dark gray shirt over the area of his right breast. "I ignored it for four months, thinking it was just a

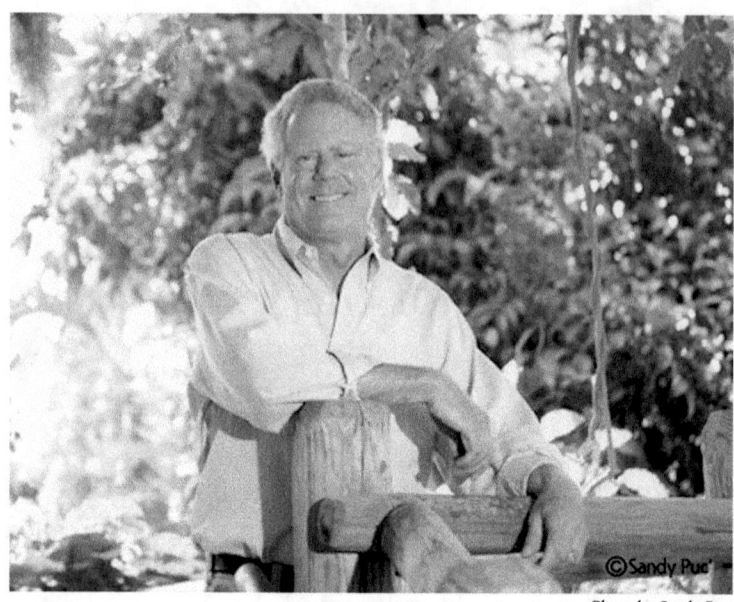

Charlie Blosten

Photo by Sandy Puc

cyst. Then I went to the doctor for something else, and I asked him to look at it. He ordered a mammogram right away and an ultrasound."

A needle biopsy followed, confirming that Charlie had an invasive ductal carcinoma. "I was shocked by the diagnosis," he said. "I could hardly comprehend how this could have happened to me."

On top of the emotional difficulty of dealing with a cancer diagnosis was the fact that his cancer was aggressive. He needed to get past the emotional jolt and get aggressive, to fight back. "I went to the Sally Jobe Breast Center in Greenwood Village," Charlie said. "The doctor recommended a mastectomy and encouraged me to have a sentinel node biopsy, which was an experimental procedure. I wanted to do whatever I could that would help me and help other people as well, so I agreed to do it.

"I was the first man to undergo the procedure," he said. "There was a group of clinicians from New Zealand who came to watch. I was awake throughout, and it *was painful*."

A total of six lymph nodes were removed from Charlie's armpit and, fortunately, all of them tested negative for cancer. Charlie's mastectomy followed the sentinel node biopsy, one hour later under general anesthesia. "My surgeon admitted that I was his first male mastectomy patient."

Even with negative nodes, an oncologist recommended chemotherapy for Charlie after the mastectomy. "I decided to fly to California for a second opinion," Charlie said, "but the opinion there was the same." Subsequently, Charlie underwent four cycles of standard chemotherapy. "I wouldn't wish that on my worst enemy," he said. "It's not fun stuff." Charlie said he felt tired and sick throughout his treatments. "I took my chemo on Thursdays so I could be back to work on Mondays and continue on with my life as much as normal," he said, "but it wasn't normal. I had nausea and constipation. I lost all of my hair, and I had no energy. I didn't want to be around people—not even my kids, who were twelve and sixteen at the time. It was summer, and they wanted to do things all the time, and I just couldn't do them."

Charlie described his first treatment as "not so bad." The second one, twenty-one days later, was "a real downer." By the third, he didn't even want to go back. He needed to take anti-anxiety medication just to get through it. Then came the fourth. "I did the last one just to get it over with."

After chemotherapy, the oncologist prescribed tamoxifen, the same hormone prescribed for women. "I didn't like it," he said. "People saw that I was moody and irritable. I stopped taking it after six months."

Charlie didn't want to wallow in worry or feel sorry for himself, so, once he was no longer in treatment, he decided he'd done everything possible to fight his cancer, and *he* was the one in control again. He became resolute to begin living his life in the best way he could. He would do something to make a difference.

"I needed a purpose in life," he said. "And now I had a cause, so five months after my surgery, I got involved with the Susan G. Komen Foundation's Race for the Cure."

The Susan G. Komen Breast Cancer Foundation was the brainchild of Nancy G. Brinker, whose sister, Suzy, had died in 1980 from breast cancer at the age of thirty-six. It was the same year my

Grandma Shaver had died from breast cancer. Because there was little community awareness at the time or support for people dealing with this killer, before her sister's death, Nancy promised Suzy she would do something to help others with the disease. Since then, with the help of thousands of people like Charlie, she has done that. Today, the foundation has raised millions for the mission of eradicating breast cancer.

Charlie began his volunteer support for the Komen Foundation along with his family. They contacted all the folks who had been so nice to him during his treatment and asked them to support him in his first Race for the Cure five-kilometer run in Denver. On the day of the race, when he saw the actual number of people involved, Charlie became aware of how big a production the Race for the Cure was. "As a lone male survivor, the Survivors Tribute at the end was too overwhelming for me to participate. There were just too many women for me to handle it, emotionally." By the end of the event, however, he had raised, $7,500—the most money of any person at the race. Charlie had made quite a statement that day, impressing upon society that, although the statistics are only one in 100,000, this disease strikes men, too.

Charlie was awarded $1,500 in gift certificates to shops in the Cherry Creek Mall. "I never used them," Charlie said. "I cashed them in and returned the money to the Race for the Cure."

Charlie continued to raise funds in the Race for the Cure for the next few years and began promoting community awareness by doing public speaking. As he became better known in the community, he was asked to give the keynote speech for the 2000 Race for the Cure survivors' pre-race reception, ten days before the race. Executives of the Saks Fifth Avenue in the Cherry Creek Mall pushed aside racks in the ladies department to make room for the cocktail party attended by more than five hundred breast cancer survivors.

"I don't remember my entire speech, but at the end I said, 'I hope you are doing your monthly self-exams because, if you're not, I will come over and do them for you.'" People laughed at

Charlie's lighthearted reminder that a simple behavior can lead to earlier detection.

Besides the Race for the Cure, Charlie became active with the Day of Caring. "I attended my first one, one year after my surgery," Charlie said. "I assume I was the only man registered. It was somewhat uncomfortable for me at first because no one seemed used to having to fit a man into this female-oriented realm. But I made up my mind I was going to sit through the workshops anyway, though I didn't go to the fashion show. I thought it wasn't for me, so I left. Then the next year, someone called and asked if I would model in the show."

Charlie was the first male model for the Day of Caring. "I got to walk into Saks Fifth Avenue and pick out whatever I wanted to wear," he said. Charlie chose a sport-coat ensemble of shirt, belt, tie, and sunglasses worth $2,000. "I came onto the stage in my own style and started getting into it. I took off my coat and strutted down the runway with it over my shoulder. Then, I walked over to Aimee Sporer, who was our mistress of ceremonies, and gave her a kiss."

Charlie was back on stage for the Day of Caring's twentieth-year celebration, where I first saw him, but he wasn't modeling that time. "I was just there for the reunion, to represent the year I modeled," he said.

Charlie didn't stop with the Race for the Cure and the Day of Caring. When he was asked to serve on the planning committee for the Komen Foundation's 4th Annual Pink Tie Affair in November 2001, he accepted that, too. This formal affair began small at its inception four years ago but has grown so large it was moved to the Pepsi Center near downtown Denver. Charlie chaired the photography committee, which had brought in Harley Davidson motorcycles to be used as the backdrop for photos for attendees who had paid $200 per ticket to enjoy the dinner, dance, and silent auction. Later, the Harleys were auctioned off along with other silent bids for items like a trip to Acapulco, an African Safari (minimum bid of $12,000), a football autographed by John Elway, and a training bike of Tour de France winner and cancer survivor, Lance

Armstrong. All the proceeds went to the Komen Foundation to pay for breast cancer screening and treatment for the low-income and uninsured population.

"It was a lot of fun," Charlie said.

"Will you do it again next year?" I asked.

"I probably will," he said.

CHAPTER 36

We Are Here

During the same month I met with Charlie, a group of us from the Association of Breast Cancer Survivors formed a team to walk in the Relay for Life that was held at the Gateway High School track in Aurora. When I met up with my teammates under our "Reach to Recovery" banner, the tight-knit group was already enjoying a social time. They were gathered on a set of movable bleachers, wearing matching purple Relay for Life survivor T-shirts with medals around their necks. White letters on the backs of their T-shirts said *I Am Here.*

Harriette and Stanley Grober stood close to the bleachers where Joyce Coville, Sally Barton, Sue Swanson, Ann Baird, Ann Hession, and Penny Cooper were sitting. Penny wore a stocking sleeve over her lymphedema arm. She always wore one and had them in different colors. This one was a pale summer blue, coordinated with her white shorts.

All of us had come to the track to promote cancer awareness and to raise funds for the American Cancer Society. Some of the other teams were busy setting up tents on the grass, where their members could sleep as they took turns walking throughout the balmy night. I got a purple shirt and joined my teammates on the bleachers, where they were busy passing around Sally Barton's *CURE* magazine. Everyone was fascinated with the new publication.

Stanley stood waiting to take our group picture while Harriette looked at the magazine. "I want a copy of the article on Chemobrain," she said, handing it back to Sally. I was unfamiliar with the magazine, which I found out was the premier edition. Out of curiosity, I would look for the magazine later as now the ladies were finally settled. Stanley smiled in a wide grin and looked into his camera. We smiled back, and he snapped the photo.

The Relay for Life ceremonies opened with an energetic martial arts performance set to music. Young boys and girls demonstrated their physical strength and discipline in routines packed with high kicks and yells. Aromas of barbeque and pizza permeated the air. Over the yelling and loud music, Anne Hession leaned toward me. "I want some of that pizza," she said. We would eat the pizza and cake, too, but first we had to take the Survivor's Victory Lap around the track.

Our Reach to Recovery group assembled first in the line of walkers on the track. Cancer survivors in purple T-shirts amassed behind us with their fellow supporters. It seemed appropriate to me that Harriette and Stanley happened to be the leaders of the whole pack. They held hands as they walked in front of Ann Hession, Joyce, and me. "I'm happy to see how good Harriette's looking," Joyce remarked, "despite her high tumor markers. My sister's are only at one hundred, and she's bald and can hardly talk."

I agreed with Joyce. Harriette did look good. "Ann," I said, "I haven't seen you since our Reach to Recovery training."

"Yes, I remember the first time I saw you," she said. "I felt sorry for you because I thought you looked so young to have breast cancer."

I got a chuckle out of that. "I'm not as young as you think. I'm almost forty-nine."

Ann said she was fifty-six and retired. "After my diagnosis I decided life is too short. So, I quit my job and never went back to work," she said. She was enjoying her life now.

At twilight hundreds of luminary bags lit our way around the track. Each one featured the name of a person who had lost his or her life to cancer or of someone who was living with cancer. Respectfully, I read the names as I walked by. "This candle is lit for Faith Witham...Nina Taylor...Jonna Hoffman...." I felt goose bumps as if I was carrying their ethereal energy with me around the track. I felt happy and alive, and I could have walked all night.

With a trail of light there is no night.

CHAPTER 37

Paranoia

Into summer, our drought worsened, and so did the fires. Much like an out-of-control cancer, they were spreading so widely that the governor declared after visiting one of the fire areas, "All of Colorado is burning." About eight fires were burning across the state. With so much ablaze, it was impossible to isolate which fire the smoke was coming from. But it didn't matter. There was just too much of it outside. The smoky haze prevailed for weeks. With the smoke from a huge fire in Arizona and another in Wyoming mingling with ours, it gave an altered impression of summer in Colorado. The gray air took away the joy in the changing of the season. People seemed to be growing used to this air, as if smoke, haze, and fire had become our way of life. I even stopped being afraid of the fires and started to unpack things I'd put in boxes, ready for a quick get away.

To add to the dismal conditions of the state, our lakes and ponds were shrinking pitifully. Everyone in Colorado was worried about the shortage of water, including Jim and me—and not just because the fires were near our home. The implications for farmers and ranchers and, therefore, all of us were becoming disastrous. They would become more so if it didn't start raining. It was depressing because there was nothing we could do but look for glimmers of hope.

Evergreen Lake offered a feeling of hope. Without any water going out over its spillway, the lake remained full. As I drove around the bend of Evergreen's Main Street on my way to work, the lake's sparkling beauty captured and comforted me. We still had *some* water.

My work that day was an interpreting assignment at a doctor's office. Waiting for the deaf patient, I switched my thoughts about the drought to an article in the *Postgraduate Medicine Journal*: "How to approach an elevated ferritin level?"

In the margin of the article, a California internist posed this question after a brief description of an actual patient case. When I scanned through the article and saw the words "serum iron," I recalled the results of the blood screen I'd had recently at the health fair. My serum iron had been elevated. All the other elements had been normal, so I hadn't been alarmed about my high iron.

But when I read further, that hyperferritinemia can be found in chronic inflammatory conditions or with *cancer*, sirens started going off in my head. I'd had a mole removed two weeks before. They said it wasn't cancer, but maybe they had missed something. Or maybe my breast cancer was back?

I had to put the journal and my concern aside when the deaf patient arrived. I was there for her. I needed to concentrate on translating *her* medical concerns to her doctor. But leaving the article unfinished left a seed of paranoia planted in my mind. When the assignment was over, I sped straight to the library. I spent the afternoon looking up the causes of high iron levels in medical journals. The articles stirred up my imagination even more. The next week I made appointments with my gynecologist and family physician to find out whether there was something wrong with me.

It was time for my annual gynecological examination anyway, I figured, and except for mammograms, I hadn't yet had any of the recommended follow-up examinations for the cancer, such as blood tests and chest X-rays. Since I'd read that routine laboratory tests and scans to detect recurrences had not made any difference in survival rates over regular mammography, I hadn't felt compelled to do them. I would have had to pay out-of-pocket for them, and since they weren't very effective at finding early cancers, I'd chosen to forgo them—up until now anyway.

"I feel fine," I told the doctors, on separate appointments, "but I want to understand why my iron levels have been creeping up over the last couple of years." I wanted to know whether I had hemochromatosis or cancer.

Neither doctor thought I had cancer or hemochromatosis. Nevertheless, they each took blood and ordered different tests. All of the test results came back showing everything was normal. I left the second doctor's office wondering whether he thought I was a hypochondriac. Meanwhile, Kim Scott called, interrupting my thoughts.

"This is a coincidence," I said. "I'm just driving past the restaurant where you and I had lunch." I didn't tell her I'd just seen the doctor because I was worried I'd had a recurrence. I was too embarrassed to admit to my paranoia over the phone. Instead, I asked whether we could get together soon, to talk about "dating issues after breast cancer."

"Dating has never been an issue for me," she said. "The only issue is my paranoia. My new boyfriend thinks I'm a hypochondriac."

"I know what you mean," I said. "We can talk about that." I understood then that paranoia about cancer returning was normal. As survivors we couldn't escape it. I hung up the phone, satisfied that I wasn't a hypochondriac. I felt better.

On my way home I stopped at the grocery store in Conifer. From the frozen food bin, I noticed Sue Niksic talking to another mom who was peering over a cart piled high with groceries and kids. Sue waved me over toward them. She was shopping without her kids.

"I've been planning to call you," I said.

Sue gave a big sigh and told me she was exhausted. "We watched fireworks at Bandimere last night, and we have company coming over tonight." She dropped her shoulders as if they were too heavy to hold up anymore. We apologized for not being in touch recently and agreed we would get together soon.

My breast cancer friends were never far from my mind. I even had dreams about them. That night, close to morning, I had one about Pat:

I am in Pat Grahn's house. It's a huge orange adobe with red concrete tile floors. The living room is spacious with a high vaulted ceiling of wood and iron crossbeams. There's a large open staircase leading up to many bedrooms on the second floor. Scores of women are in the house, where they have gathered for some kind of religious meeting. I am here to talk to Pat. I want to know how she's doing, but she is too busy with the other women to talk to me. I'm surprised to see a lighted Christmas tree in her house, in the middle of July.

I woke to the sound of water dripping, conscious of the fact that Pat didn't live in an adobe house with red concrete tile floors and I that I must have been dreaming. It was 6:00 A.M. and not yet light. From my bed I could see mist outside through the window in the next room. I wondered whether it was raining. When I got a better look, I saw it was indeed. The ground was soaked, and I smiled, thinking perhaps this was the end of the drought—and the end to the fires. Recalling my dream, I resolved to call Pat.

I called her that day, but it would actually be another couple of months before we were able to see each other. In the meantime a couple of unexpected events happened. First, I stumbled upon the website for the Susan G. Komen Foundation. The foundation said it had a library named after Judge Linda Palmieri. Since my breast cancer diagnosis, I hadn't been thinking much about Linda Palmieri or the day I'd stood dumbfounded in her courtroom when I learned of her death. But now, seeing her name as a member of the sisterhood, I felt a new connection with her. I would never be able to tell Linda Palmieri I was a sister, too, but at least I could go to her library.

I had it pictured as something spectacular—a beautiful and shining glass building, full of books. Unfortunately, on the website I found no mention as to the location of this library, and there was no explanation of how it came to be named after her. I was determined to find out.

It took me a few weeks to track down the new location of the Susan G. Komen Foundation. I finally learned their Denver office had moved to the Mullen Building at 1895 Franklin, an old brick building next to St. Joseph's Hospital. The person who answered the phone didn't know anything about the Linda Palmieri Library, but she thought the office had some books to lend. She said I was welcome to stop by. A few weeks later I got that opportunity.

I was disappointed that there was no shining glass building, but I was still eager to find out how the library came to be named after Judge Palmieri. It was obvious other people besides me had thought highly of her, and I hoped someone there could tell me. I found a young woman working in the small upstairs office. When I inquired about the library, she led me to a small room one door down the hall. The library consisted of about forty books and half as many videotapes arranged in two standup bookshelves. Sadly, the young woman didn't know how the library got its name. Nevertheless, I left happy with four borrowed books and the name and phone number of the former director. Maybe she could tell me who named the library.

CHAPTER 38

Musical Chairs

―――――◆―――――

"When I go, I will go fighting."
Harriette Grober, at Spa for the Spirit, 1997

Contacting the former director of the Susan G. Komen Foundation only resulted in disappointment when I kept reaching an answering machine. In actuality I was inching toward finding out what I wanted to know—it just wasn't the time yet. In the interim, something else came unexpectedly—a downpour of rain. Having been in drought mode for so long, the amount of water that came with this storm was unforeseen. I was unlucky to be downtown shopping the evening the storm hit.

I pulled out from the store's covered garage, shocked to find the street's intersection flooded. My sweeping wipers couldn't keep up with the amount of water streaming down my windshield, and it fogged over instantly. I used a tissue to clear a circle of mist away, only to discover that the streets up ahead were also flooded.

My arms began to shake at the steering wheel as I willed my Subaru through two and a half feet of rushing water. I couldn't believe this was really happening. There was so much water I feared being suddenly swept away, into a dangerous river flowing right through downtown Denver. I looked for a safe place to pull over, but there was no place without rushing water. I was afraid I was going to die this way. I prayed the blue Volkswagen bug in front of me didn't stall or float off sideways before we could both get through to safety.

Luckily, or miraculously, my Subaru seemed to swim like a horse because safety didn't come for eight more blocks. A half hour later, the storm and the water subsided and disappeared as quickly as they had come. The pounding of my heart subsided much more slowly.

This frightful experience was just a memory the next morning. The surprise downpour had cleared the smoky haze from the air, but it was to be another hot, dry day in spite of the rain the evening before. Already it was heating up when I arrived at the Cancer Center a little before noon. Shortly after came Harriette. In white shorts, she looked cooler than I in my long skirt. I'd come from work to be with her.

"You're early," she said, signing in at the desk. "I have to see the doctor first. I'm having trouble with my left leg again."

I nodded and eased into a chair in the waiting room. I watched her walk down the hall to see whether she was limping, but I couldn't detect anything. She veered around the corner and disappeared behind a man who was talking loudly to a small woman hunched over in a wheelchair. Dressed in purple pants, a pink straw hat, and high-top tennis shoes, it was hard to tell her age. The man, who I assumed was her son, lifted her stiff frail body and pushed her farther back into her seat. He adjusted her sweater and her hat, all while her body never changed its position. "Are you okay?" he asked, moving his face close to hers to hear her answer. "Why, why?" he said, raising his voice as if that would make her speak louder. I felt sad for the two of them, wondering what affliction she was suffering from. Cancer metastasized to her brain? Whatever it was, it seemed horribly difficult for both of them.

Harriette reappeared, after seeing Dr. Hinshaw. "My numbers didn't go up," she said. "There's just the stubborn spot in the femur. We have to radiate again, for the pain." I acknowledged her statement with a look of concern as I followed her to a chemotherapy treatment room. Another young couple was already settled into the semi-private room. The woman and her husband looked to be in their early thirties. I wondered whether she had breast cancer, too.

While the nurse drew blood from the port to check Harriette's Protime (the blood clotting time), Harriette showed us the scab on her knee from her three-week-old bicycle accident. She had injured her ring finger, too. "They almost had to cut my ring off," she said. "That upset me more than the stitches in my knee." Actually, Harriette was more concerned today about Stanley. He seemed more confused than usual. She was also worrying because her long-term disability insurance company was filing for bankruptcy. "And they're doing mold and air quality tests at our house today. I hope we pass because we need to move out of the hotel soon."

With her husband standing nearby, the young woman sat next to an IV pole unfolding a shiny, quilted foil square. She placed it over her head like a hat. Her husband helped her cover it with a towel, which made her look like Little Red Riding Hood. I'd read that, for some lower-dose chemotherapies, using ice on the scalp during treatments could prevent hair loss. Harriette must not have known this because she asked the woman what the foil pack was for.

"It's a cold pack," she answered. "Supposedly, if you start it fifteen minutes before infusion and keep it on during and after for a little bit, it works to keep your hair."

"I've never lost my hair," Harriette bragged, "but some people in my support group drank a special tea to prevent theirs from falling out. I just pat mine dry, very carefully, after I wash it."

We found out the young woman was receiving chemotherapy for lupus, and it seemed to be working. When Harriette told her she'd been on 5-FU every week for ten years, for metastatic breast cancer, she seemed interested. "...[U]ntil last December, when it stopped working," Harriette said. "Now, I'm on Taxotere." I guessed the woman didn't know how to respond because she said nothing more.

Harriette and I went back to visiting until the nurse returned an hour later, when the bag of Taxotere was empty. She snapped open the yellow plastic clip, designed to prevent nurses from sticking themselves, and released the needle from Harriette's port. Free from the pole, we were on our way.

We lunched outdoors at a Mexican café. Harriette had already decided today to tell me about the Spa for the Spirit. I munched on a chicken burrito while she picked at her salad and reminisced about her experience at the four-day mountain retreat for women with advanced breast cancer. She had attended the first Spa for the Spirit Retreat in June of 1997. "I was reluctant to go at first because I didn't like leaving Cyndi alone for a whole weekend," Harriette said. "But I got a flyer in the mail about it, saying it was at a conference center on a beautiful mountain ranch, so it seemed like a good thing to try.

"A group of us rode down on a charter bus that left from a hospital in Denver. There were thirteen of us, plus the staff. I sat down on the bus next to a woman who was bald. She introduced herself and told me she was a judge. Immediately, I felt intimidated. I didn't think I'd be smart enough to converse with a judge, but she was a wonderful woman."

"A judge?" I asked, instantly flashing back to the day when Magistrate Vance told me what had happened to Judge Palmieri. "Was she Linda Palmieri?"

"Yes. She died shortly after our retreat."

"I knew her," I said. "I worked in her courtroom a number of times." Again, I felt the sadness of her loss, yet the sadness was tinged with a good feeling knowing that Harriette had known her, too. "She *was* a wonderful person," I agreed. I asked Harriette whether she knew about the library named after her. She wasn't aware of it.

"Linda and I talked about a lot of things on the bus," Harriette said. "I found her fascinating and a delight. She got sick while we were at the retreat. She had to go to the hospital in Colorado Springs, and then she came back in a wheelchair. We all felt bad for her."

I was still thinking of Linda Palmieri as Harriette went on to describe the place where they had gone. The chartered bus had taken them to The Nature Place, affiliated with the Western Camps in Florissant, Colorado. At tree line the women got off the bus and set foot on the ranch's six thousand acres. A vast green meadow filled with wildflowers and a sparkling pond spread before them. "It was so beautiful, it gave me goose bumps," Harriette said. She caught the scent of the pine forest intermingled with aspen groves, where there were boulders to climb and trails to hike. Majestic Pikes Peak towered over the ranch off to the east. "The ranch was owned by an uncle of one of the ten Spa for the Spirit founders, a woman who also had breast cancer. I remember that woman's energy and her sense of humor. She had a great positive attitude despite cancer in her brain. She was an inspiration to us all."

While Harriette remembered the people she'd met at the Spa for the Spirit, we were heating up in the sun. Our table was the only one in the row without an umbrella. All of the other tables had been occupied when we brought our lunch outside. Though I was melting, I tried to ignore it.

Harriette didn't seem to notice the heat. "We stayed in little cabins there," she continued. Each wood cabin had a stone fireplace with a rustic ambience and an outside viewing deck. Designed for double occupancy, they had full baths and sitting rooms that provided them with all the comforts of home, save for a telephone and a television. "Each of us had a roommate because they didn't want us to ever be alone, but I didn't spend too much time with my roommate. I spent more time with a thirty-year-old woman who had inflammatory breast cancer. She had a four-year-old child at home. She was Egyptian, young looking, dark skinned, and beautiful. She wore blue jeans, and since she was bald, she wore a baseball cap with a black ponytail sewn in. We became friends right away.

"I met others I became friends with, too. One, who I'll never forget, said to me when she learned I'd just quit work, 'When one door closes, another one opens, but the halls are a bitch.' Gloria Kubel, who I'd known since 1984 was there, too, leading Yoga and Tai Chi exercises.

"During the weekend some of the women hiked, and we ate from a gourmet, vegan soy-menu. We had meetings where we discussed topics related to coping with late-stage cancer. "You couldn't hide in your denial there," Harriette said. "Every discussion and activity was meant to be healing. We had therapeutic massages and group singing."

Once, they lay together on their backs on a wooden deck. With a "giant singing bowl" at their heads and their feet pointing away, they looked like human spokes around its hub. "As one person rubbed the rim of the bowl, you could hear a deep humming. It sent relaxing, singing vibrations traveling all through your body. You could actually experience balancing, healing effects. I've never felt anything like it."

In art therapy the women made Didgeridoos—cylinders through which sound travels, like what the native Australian aborigines used for communication. "We painted them and put nails inside and created music."

The women learned about the Lakota Indians, who would go into battle, and when they came out victorious, they would decorate "Coup Sticks." Each time the Indians returned alive from another battle, they would add more decorations of feathers, paint, and leather strips to their "Coup Sticks." The warriors with the most decorated sticks had come through the most battles. The women designed "Coup Sticks" of their own to tell their stories.

"I'm not into stuff like glue and paint," Harriette said. "I'm not very creative. Usually, I avoid any kind of arts and crafts, but I got into the feathers, and I made a 'power stick.' Because I think of myself as timid and shy, it represented my strength. Then we made a timeline of different stages we've been through in our lives. On a huge sheet of paper, we drew pictures and wrote phrases about our hard times as well as our fun times.

"I was most excited about my stick. When I came home, I showed it to Cyndi and Stanley. I still have it hanging in my living room. But Cyndi got angry that day when she saw my timeline. 'You've only had fun with Jeff,' she cried. I'd just come home feeling euphoric, and then we had a big fight over that timeline. All my euphoria was ruined, and I took the timeline and ripped it up." Harriette regretted later she'd done that.

"I was a pioneer for Spa for the Spirit," she continued, "like I am for a lot of the breast cancer programs. We used to have reunions for it, but I quit going to them. They were depressing because I made friends with those women and then they started dying. I felt like I was playing musical chairs with them. Sandy was one I had really connected with at the retreat, and we stayed friends after that. She was in remission. But one day we were supposed to go to a coalition meeting together, and she called and said she didn't feel well. Shortly after that she went into a hospice. We were friends until the very end."

Harriette showed little emotion except for a few times when her voice got quiet and she paused. "My friend with the inflammatory breast cancer turned down a bone marrow transplant a year or so after the retreat. She hadn't wanted any heavy-duty chemotherapy. Later, she decided she wanted the transplant, but by then she was ineligible. Instead, she tried an alternative treatment in Arizona, but then she died in 1999."

Hearing Harriette talk about the friends she'd lost was heartrending for me. Sometimes, survivors feel guilty about having survived when friends haven't, but Harriette didn't seem to feel that. She seemed sad but also a little angry that her friends had died. "I'm one of the last two women still around from that group," she added. "I still have the T-shirt everyone signed at the end of that weekend. She smiled then, remembering the bittersweet times and wonderful friendships she'd made. "That's how I know how many people have crossed over to the other side."

As I imagined what memories and emotions that T-shirt held, Harriette and I walked back to our cars. In the sisterhood we were all pulling for one another, and it was hard losing even one. I hoped never to lose Harriette to the other side, but if it happened, I wanted to be there to make the crossing a little easier. For Grandma Shaver there had been no Spa for the Spirit and no one to support her in crossing over. I was glad that the Spa for the Spirit had been there for Linda Palmieri. Somehow, I felt closer to her.

CHAPTER 39

She's Talking Months

Nothing much improved in the week following the downpour. The temperature hung in the nineties, the drought remained unrelenting, and another fire had ignited in the mountains near Estes Park. Things for Harriette weren't improving either, yet she hung in there with dogged determination.

It was July 18th, and I was waiting for her in the lobby at the Rocky Mountain Cancer Center. Three women sat across from me, absorbed in an exchange. One of the women was bald and wore a white straw hat. I heard her talking to the others. "I have a tumor in my chest," she was saying. "It's bone cancer." My attention turned to Harriette, who had just walked in with a paperback book tucked under her arm titled *Don't Sweat the Small Stuff*. When she sat down next to me, she recognized two of the women who'd been talking and were now walking toward us. I didn't know how or from where Harriette knew them, but it appeared that people in the cancer world all seemed to know each other. "How're you doing?" one of them asked her.

"Not good," Harriette said. "Stanley's neurological report says he has frontal lobe deterioration, and I'm having a hard time getting things regulated with my chemotherapy this month. I can't live with this pain in my left hip."

The woman told Harriette she was being treated for an eye infection, a side effect of her chemotherapy treatment. Her eyes were swollen so badly that she was looking out from small slits.

Harriette got up from her chair and walked away from us. "I'm going to find out from Dr. Hinshaw how bad my bone scan is."

The woman who'd been talking to Harriette sat down and started telling me about her side effects from Rituxan, the treatment she'd had that put her B-Cell non-Hodgkin's Lymphoma into remission. It seemed that people really needed to talk about their cancer—so much so that they talked to strangers about it. As the woman began complaining about western medicine, Harriette beckoned me from the end of the hall. She wanted me to join her in the examination room, where she had just seen Dr. Hinshaw.

"It's bad," Harriette said. She was talking fast. "The Taxotere's not working, and I have a new spot on my left temple. She's talking months!"

"Months?" I repeated, wondering what she meant. I needed Harriette. A few months left for her to live was not acceptable. She was my inspiration, my friend, my role model in how to overcome obstacles. Harriette's work was not done. We had a mission. We had a book to write, and she had others who needed her. She had to find a place for Cyndi.

Dr. Hinshaw had said originally that Harriette would be on Taxotere for six months. Now, two months later, she wanted Harriette to go on AC, Adriamycin, and Cytoxan, the regimen normally used as a first-line treatment. She said there was nothing more she could offer. "I'm not going to make it, am I?" Harriette had asked.

"Well, there is no cure," Dr. Hinshaw answered.

Harriette talked while she and I waited for the oncology nurse who would come to explain the new chemotherapy treatment. "Last week, when Jeff gave me a bear hug after our evening ride, I asked him if he could see the lights. He said, 'What lights?' I was seeing circles of colors: red, orange, green, and blue colors around car headlights. I saw them again last night. I'm scared," she said. "I'm scared I won't be around to take care of Cyndi."

I took her hand. My eyes filled with tears. "I'm scared, too," I said. "How can I help you?"

"Write the book," she said.

After we moved to another room with a bed, a nurse came in carrying a consent form and a packet of information about the side effects of AC. She started to hand Harriette a couple of booklets, when Harriette interrupted, "I've been a cancer patient since 1984. I know all about those books."

Harriette just wanted to know whether constipation was going to be a side effect. "I already have a problem with that."

The nurse sat behind the bedside table, speaking in a soft and serious manner while Harriette and I sat on the bed. "The drugs will cause the platelets and white cell count to drop around day eight, nine, or ten," she said. "Day fourteen will be the lowest, and you can expect fever, aches, and chills. Then the counts will start to come up, and you'll have a week to recover before the next treatment on day twenty-one. If the counts go too low, we have Neupogen or Neulasta injections to cover you through the low point. Later, the red cell count may drop, too, and cause anemia.

"You'll lose your hair," she continued, "and the chemotherapy could cause mouth sores. For this, you can rinse with 1/4 tsp baking soda in six ounces of warm water mixed with 1/8 tsp salt. You may also experience fatigue."

I looked over at Harriette and saw the words "Bryce Canyon" printed on the sleeve of her maroon T-shirt. A souvenir from one of her bike trips, I assumed. She finally responded to the nurse. "I can't have fatigue," Harriette said. "I take care of a very sick daughter, and I help my son with his business. Am I going to be too tired to ride my bike thirty miles?"

"Well, you'll need to keep a thermometer with you at all times because, with a low count, you probably won't get the same symptoms to alert you to an infection as you normally would. And you must keep nourishing protein snacks with you."

"I'm a carb person," Harriette said.

The nurse enumerated (or specified) foods that should not be eaten, like raw or unwashed vegetables or unpasteurized cheese because of organisms that might get past a weakened immune system. "Scrub them well," she warned, "or only eat bananas and oranges. And don't be around any fresh flowers."

Silently, I observed their exchange, catching a few of Harriette's sidelong glances toward me. I felt increasingly anxious and quite overwhelmed by the time the nurse began explaining how Harriette should take the anti-nausea medications she already had displayed on the table—Anzemet and Decadron.

Harriette looked visibly upset. "Steroids make me hungry and gain weight. I don't want to gain weight, and my daughter has severe side effects from steroids."

"The Decadron makes the Anzemet work better," the nurse said. "You can take four milligrams of Decadron with breakfast to control nausea and vomiting. We're hitting you hard with the chemotherapy, so we're using a multi-attack to control the nausea." There were also Ativan and a generic Compazine she could take at 2:00 A.M. or as needed.

Harriette was aghast. "I don't want any drugs that are going to make me mentally unsharp."

The two of them got into a debate over the drugs and the times Harriette should take them, but the nurse was adamant. She then added a few more instructions about sunscreen and sitz baths should the chemotherapy cause skin breakdowns in the perineal area. I hoped Harriette was keeping all the information straight because I'd gotten lost at about the time the nurse mentioned 2:00 A.M. medications. I wondered how anyone could manage all of this, especially if she was sick. If it were me, I think I would have walked out of the room at that point.

I had elected to keep quiet during their conversation, but now I felt obliged to say something. "Maybe you could write down the schedule for her nausea medicines and label that bottle of generic compazine," I said to the nurse. I pointed to the little white bottle she had in front of her. "Not for you, Harriette—for Stanley, in case he has to get the medicine for you," I suggested. I knew she was very organized as far as her family's medications, keeping hers in the linen closet, Stanley's in the kitchen, and Cyndi's in a huge cart; however, I was worried about what would happen if she became too ill to manage them herself.

"Will I get short of breath?" Harriette asked the nurse. "And what about heart symptoms, and how long will it work?"

The nurse admitted she didn't know how long the AC would work. This was uncharted territory. AC was usually used as a first-line treatment, and as far as Dr. Hinshaw knew, as a third-line treatment the longest it had worked was three months. But the nurse assured Harriette they were not trying to slow her down. "You can call anytime with questions or concerns," she said.

Without knowing that one Anzemet pill cost between $35–40, Harriette expressed concern about the cost of the medications. "I have a $1,000-per-year prescription limit," she said. By this time Harriette seemed reluctant, yet was resigned to take the AC. She reached for her water bottle and took a long gulp. "I'll do it for Cyndi," she said.

Another nurse had already prepared Harriette's first dose of the red Adriamycin and administered it through the port as Harriette signed the consent form. After the nurses left, Harriette lay on the bed with her head propped up on a pillow. The clear Cytoxan was already dripping from the IV pole. I asked her if she was okay.

"I'm all right for right now, but I don't know if I'm going to be here next year," she said. "Jeff may need to find somebody else to help him. Stanley asked me if I wanted him to come with me today, and I told him I would be okay because you were going to be here."

That touched me. I was glad I could be with her. I asked Harriette whether she had been reluctant to sign the form. "No," she said, "signing that form only means I've been given the information, not that I am agreeing to take it." She was in disbelief that things had come to this. "I exercise, I take care of myself, and now I'm putting this garbage into my body!"

I hadn't been prepared for this change in events either, and I had to clarify one thing. "What did you mean when you said Dr. Hinshaw is talking months?"

"That's how long she said I'd be on the AC, not how long I have to live."

Though greatly relieved, I worried about Harriette for the next two days, wondering whether she was too sick to take care of Cyndi. I phoned her twice but couldn't reach her. Several days later she told me she'd been out riding her bike over the weekend and had decided to go against Dr. Hinshaw's advice. "I've quit the AC," she said. "I'm an athlete, and I'm not going to be sick while its good biking weather."

CHAPTER 40

A Second and a Third Opinion

Harriette had quit the AC but was still on Zometa for her bones and Faslodex, the new hormone we'd heard raves about at the Day of Caring. Harriette told me she hadn't liked the flu-like symptoms caused by the AC and the burning pain it caused in her legs, *and* she didn't like that she couldn't eat salads while on this strong chemotherapy. "What am I supposed to eat?" she wondered. "Where's my quality of life on this drug?" I didn't know what to say to her. She used me as her sounding board anyway. In the sisterhood, this was where we got our grounding. Without it, we were left floating.

She knew her disease was progressing now, and her options were drying up. She'd had nine and a half years of 5-FU, and now it seemed her tumors were resistant to it. "Maybe I should go back on the 5-FU again, but at a higher dose," she said. "Xeloda." It was a pill, available since 1998, which converted to 5-FU and was more convenient to take than intravenous 5-FU. A side effect of the high-dose oral medication, however, was hand-foot syndrome, in which the skin of her palms and the soles of her feet could become dry, swollen, and cracked.[1] To add to her worries, Harriette was concerned that Medicare didn't cover oral prescriptions. "Perhaps it won't be covered, and Xeloda won't be an option anyway."

One decision was easy. Harriette decided she definitely didn't want radiation. It weakened the area of the tumor, and she didn't want anything that might cause weak legs. "Maybe I'll just get through the biking season and our anniversary trip to Washington, D.C., and then I can start again on AC in the winter," she said.

At the same time she kept hearing in her mind "hormones, hormones, hormones"—the words of the oncology expert at the Day of Caring. He had said it was better to exhaust all of the hormonal treatments first, since they were usually effective for a period of time and had fewer side effects, and to save the harsh chemotherapies for last. Harriette would do whatever she had to, to live, but in the meantime she was seeking a second opinion and a third and talking to Dr. Garfield, who was retired now. I hoped she would hear what she wanted to hear.

She did. Thursday evening, July 25th, I was starting to cook dinner when Harriette called, very excited with the news. With her family by her side, through lingering mouth sores, a numb tongue, and thinning hair, she had consulted Dr. Jotte, a young oncologist who had worked at the university for five years and was now a partner at the Rocky Mountain Cancer Center. "It's an absolute miracle you're still here," he told her. "You're looking for quality time now."

Harriette was thrilled that Dr. Jotte agreed to do as Dr. Garfield had always done: to follow her pain and not her tumor markers. The blood tests for tumor activity were not always perfect in indicating what was going on with the cancer. For now, he said he would keep her on Faslodex and Zometa and she could use Advil to control pain. If necessary, he would put her back on Taxotere. It was what she wanted. Harriette was happy. For now, we could all be happy with the game plan, but no one could predict how long things would stay this way or when she'd be forced to choose her last move.

Days after our phone conversation, I flipped through the pages of the *Rocky Mountain News* while I waited for Harriette at a Perkins restaurant. A picture of a young swimming instructor, teaching the last lesson of the season to five splashing children, reminded me of the many summers I'd taught swimming lessons. The caption under the photo read: "The city will take the 185,000 gallons of water to irrigate parks, playing fields and medians suffering during the drought." The city of Aurora was responding creatively to the need to conserve water. It planned to transfer the water in all of the city's outdoor pools into tank trucks, dechlorinate the water, and then reuse it to water areas that otherwise wouldn't be watered due to mandatory restrictions. These were dire straits. Like Harriette's options for drugs, the city's water sources were drying up, as was our little stream at home. I was glad I didn't have a lawn to worry about like the people in Aurora. Our home sat among pine trees. I only had to worry about fire.

But I wasn't really focused on fire. I was eager to see Harriette, as she and Jeff had just returned from their annual bike trip to Aspen. They'd been going there since 1996, and Harriette wasn't going to let hip pain, thinning hair, and mouth sores stop her from going this year either.

"It was touch and go up until it was time to leave," she said as we lunched on chicken and mozzarella cheese sandwiches. "The chemotherapy had thrown me for a loop, and my leg pain was so bad I thought I had a fracture." She'd been lifting Cyndi a great deal and wondered whether that might have caused one. But the doctor told her that her bones were blastic now, strong, not lytic and brittle as they might have been without Aredia. "The doctor thinks I'm at low risk for a fracture, so we decided to go ahead with our plans. Getting ready for every trip is like that for us. Usually, it's something with Cyndi."

Cyndi often got sick right before they were scheduled to leave. Once, they'd had to cancel a trip, and another time Cyndi got so sick she almost required a tracheotomy to breathe. They started to believe the episodes were brought on purely by an emotional reaction to being left behind. But this time it was something with Stanley. "He got a blood clot in his leg, and I had to take him to the hospital. He's okay now."

Harriette and Jeff went on their way and the first day were able to bike thirty-nine miles along the path of Glenwood Canyon. It took them three hours and was the first time in years they'd biked there without any rain. "I was surprised my stamina was so good," she said. "We did a lot of high-fives." After the first night in

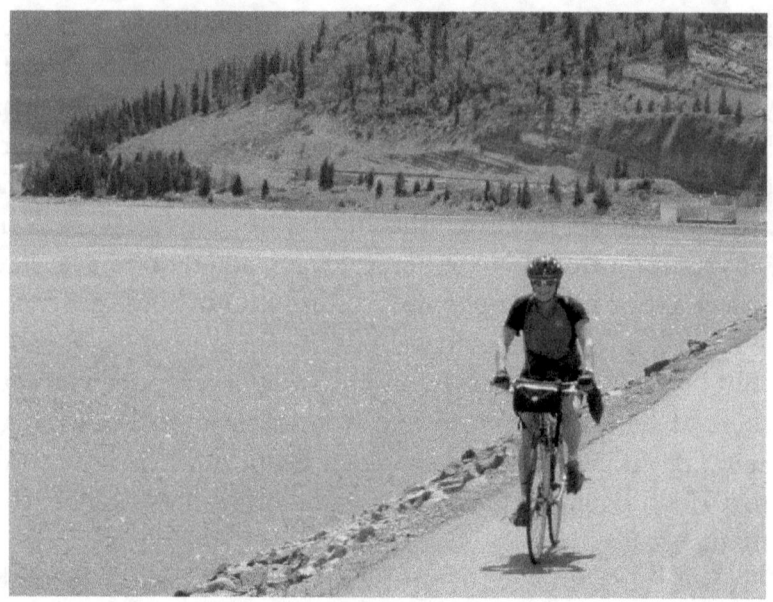

Harriette, biking in Glenwood Springs, Colorado, 2004.

Glenwood Springs, they drove to Aspen and took a gondola ride to the top of Aspen Mountain for the annual music festival. Harriette remembered how it had poured rain on them the year before. There was no rain this year. They were able to sit on a blanket and enjoy a vegetarian pizza while they listened to the music. Later, they went on another bike ride. "We rode nine miles and stopped because of heavy gravel on the path. We changed clothes in a gas station in town and went to an art gallery instead." Afterward, they shared some ice cream.

Harriette was elated that they'd been able to do so much, and she didn't leave out any details. I was envious of their trip. With a guided hike, great food, and lovely weather, it sounded relaxing and heavenly, including the horseback riding, which Harriette admitted she didn't like. "I hate heights," she said. "I'm out of my comfort zone on horses. The horse was the one in control, and he knew it." Harriette had felt the same way when she rode a horse in Bryce Canyon down a very narrow track. But they ended their fun with something she was comfortable with: another bike ride, from Breckenridge to Frisco, topped off with more ice cream.

Harriette was looking forward to the Moonlight Classic next. The twenty-mile night ride through the streets of Denver raised money for Seniors Inc. "We start at the state capital. There's a mass of bikes, music, and food every five miles…and pancakes." Harriette loved pancakes.

As I sipped my iced tea, I remembered the day I met Harriette at the American Cancer Society. As I had reached out, so had she. Since then, we'd come a long way together and built a friendship. I asked her something that had been on my mind since then. "In the beginning, why were you so willing to tell me your story, and what made you trust me so quickly?"

"Everybody always told me I should write a book. If you tell your story, your life will carry on. I hope my story will help other people to cope with adversity. I trusted you because you were a breast cancer survivor."

CHAPTER 41

Spa for the Spirit

Some matters I can't let go of until I've resolved them. I'm not comfortable leaving things unfinished or having questions go unanswered. If I'm curious about something, I investigate it. If I start a project, I finish it. If I have questions, I keep searching until I find answers. Sometimes the answers are a long time in coming. Other times, they come quickly or in unpredictable ways. I got answers one day when I met Pat Crawford, the director of the Spa for the Spirit. I found out how the Linda Palmieri Library came to be.

Ever since Harriette had told me about Spa for the Spirit, I'd wanted to learn more about this healing place. And so, on another sweltering day in September, I talked with Pat Crawford in her office. She was a small, quiet-mannered woman. "We've just moved in here," she said, which explained why the room looked so stark and empty even with two brand new desks and chairs. A few books neatly arranged in a shelf provided the only warmth in the decor.

After I mentioned that I was friends with Harriette Grober and that I'd known Linda Palmieri, both of whom had participated in the inaugural Spa for the Spirit retreat in 1997, Pat remembered fondly, "Ah, yes, Harriette," she said, smiling. "There aren't many around like her. She is one of the longest survivors of metastatic breast cancer I know."

When she paused, I thought perhaps Pat was going to explain why Harriette had been able to defy the odds for so long and still be with us, but she didn't. Pat couldn't explain why. She only knew there's power in living with purpose, something she had learned from the many women who had come to Spa for the Spirit.

However quiet and soft-spoken she seemed at first, Pat soon enlivened the stark room with a voice overflowing with emotion. As she spoke of these women, she revealed her understanding of life and of death.

Pat described how she began working with the Spa for the Spirit. She had been a breast cancer nurse specialist when she and a group of stage IV breast cancer survivors and several cancer care professionals came up with the idea for the retreat. "Three of the founders were young women with metastatic breast cancer," Pat said. "They felt like the medical community had given up on them after they had failed medical treatments."

Similar to how Harriette felt in 1992 when she'd been told she had only six months to two years to live, and again in 1994, when her friends from the coalition didn't think she should be secretary because they "didn't think she was gonna make it," these women with stage IV cancer were treated like they had "Dead Woman Walking" signs printed across their foreheads.

"They felt like they didn't belong in support groups because they had to censor what they said, to protect the women with early-stage cancers," Pat continued. "They said, 'We are everybody's worst nightmare. There's nothing just for us.' So we wanted to provide an opportunity where women with advanced cancer could nurture their spirits and focus on hope and being alive."

Spa for the Spirit aimed to rejuvenate the body, mind, and spirit through music, gentle exercise, art, massage, and meditation. Pat couldn't talk about the program without speaking individually of some of the two hundred women she had met during the last five years. To her, each one seemed remarkable and brave.

"In their day-to-day lives, they're busy, and they stuff their stress and emotions," she said. "When they come to the retreat, they're not looking for telephones and places to hook up their computers. They're looking to get in touch with nature and reconnect with their inner spirits. I see them become relaxed and begin to build trust among themselves. They feel safe, and then they're able to get deeply in touch with their own hearts and spirits. Then the 'stuff' starts to bubble out. They talk and they cry. No subject is off limits because the others know what they're talking about. They're living it also."

The women share their most intimate fears and thoughts, and they ask the hard questions they can't ask anyone else, not the doctors who are treating them or their families, who think they're being morbid. "We don't shy away from talking about fears of dying and death. Here, it's safe to talk about those things. They ask graphic and practical questions like: How am I going to die? What will it feel like? What happens to my body after I die?" Through guided imagery, Pat leads the women in visualizing their own deaths. To help them get over their fear, she guides them to choreograph their own journey.

Although I was not living with stage IV metastatic breast cancer, I had the same curiosity as the women at the Spa for the Spirit. I wanted to know the answers to these questions, too. I told Pat about my grandmother's death from breast cancer and how my mother had said Grandma had died from fluid on her lungs. I felt comfortable asking Pat the questions I'd wondered about for a long time. "What does a person with breast cancer actually die from? Is it from fluid on the lungs? What causes that?"

"It's different for each person," she said. "No one can predict exactly how the death will occur. It can be a totally unexpected crisis, like a sudden blood clot, or the lungs just give out. Or the death can be a result of the actual cancer in the liver or the brain or the lungs."

The liver is a vital organ. Since it is the waste warehouse, if it becomes cancerous, it can no longer do its job of cleaning toxins out of the body, and the result is fatal. In the lungs there are two sacs surrounding them that normally have no space between them, but when there's an injury or cancer, the sacs can come apart. Then the cancer cells draw fluid in, in what's referred to as *malignant pleural effusion*. It used to be common that people died from this, but now doctors have advanced techniques for treating it. It's a less common cause of death.

Although this wasn't a cheerful topic, I felt less fearful understanding this physiology. Pat reminded me that many long-term survivors have only metastasis to their bones, which is painful but not necessarily fatal. That explained somewhat why Harriette was a long-term survivor and gave me comfort knowing we might have a longer time to enjoy her.

I understood, too, that Grandma must have been suffering from malignant pleural effusion when she died. In my mind I saw her lying in her hospital bed and remembered her last words to me. Through morphine and labored breathing she'd whispered, "I'm sooo happy. I'm so happy you came." I kissed her goodbye. The next day Mom told me Grandma had passed away during the night. I was glad her suffering was over but sad that she'd died alone.

I didn't tell Pat Crawford of my daydream just then. I didn't think she'd want to know the sad details of my last visit with Grandma. She had probably experienced the deaths of many women. Besides, she was practically glowing thinking of the remarkable women at the Spa for the Spirit. It was clear that these women had brought her much joy. "I see these women change so much from Thursday to Sunday," she said. "They blossom in just four days, given the nourishment of unconditional love from eighteen other people that they never knew before. It's a great gift to give women, and I get so much back."

Pat remembered Linda Palmieri as someone who had especially stood out. "I met Linda for the first time on the bus as we boarded that Thursday afternoon. Right away, I was struck by her. Most of us were in T-shirts and shorts, but Linda had on a leopard print dress and pill-box hat. She had a strong presence."

Pat recalled that Linda had begun experiencing excruciating pain in her leg and that they'd tried to help alleviate it. When they couldn't, they'd had to take her to the hospital. "In the emergency room they were able to get her pain under control, and then we got her back to camp at five o'clock in the morning. Later, all of the women crowded around Linda in her wheelchair. She'd just been through a night of hell, and she announced, 'I feel incredible peace and love. The peace in my core is pervasive.'"

Hearing about Linda, I felt the hairs rise on my arms. The power of the sisterhood filled us with this strength and peace. It brought me to tears.

Linda had the goal to live for just two more events in her life: to attend the first Spa for the Spirit Retreat and to see the birth of her grandchild. After she came back from the hospital, she made it through the rest of the retreat. Soon after, she was in the hospital again, at the same time and place where her grandson was born. Linda was able to bond with the baby, accomplishing her one last goal before she passed away a week later.

Pat Crawford had known Linda Palmieri for only a very short time at the end of her life, though when she heard Linda had passed away, she attended a gathering in her honor at the courthouse in Jefferson County, where Linda had worked. It was held in the building known as the "Taj Mahal" for its gold dome.

"Each paralegal and judge told stories about her energy and her kindness," Pat said. "Each story was better than the first, and everyone expressed how much she would be missed. Then, Tomiko Takeda, the president of the board of directors of the Susan G. Komen Foundation, announced they had received a contribution from Linda's family, requesting the money be used for a breast cancer library in her name."

I missed Linda Palmieri as well. I wished I'd known about the memorial service, so I could have attended and said goodbye to her. But knowing now how the library at the Susan G. Komen Foundation had been named was my way of saying goodbye. I'd learned the answer to my question, and I felt elated, like I had discovered the pot of gold at the end of the rainbow.

Pat Crawford had never had cancer, but she understood us. She helped us understand things in a way others couldn't, in a way that brought us peace. Pat loaned me an album of photos from the first retreat and gave me a picture of Harriette on the bus, waving goodbye to The Nature Place staff. It is a picture I will cherish forever.

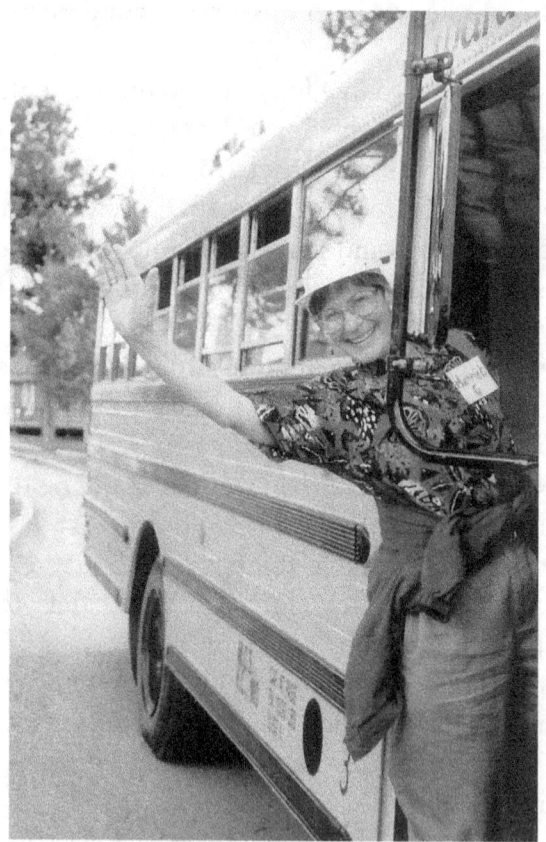

Harriette, at Spa for the Spirit.

CHAPTER 42

Friends, Biopsies, Scares, and Loss

October was Breast Cancer Awareness month. On my way to the Cherry Creek Shopping Center to see the mall's annual exhibit promoting this theme, I was thinking about Harriette. She'd been ecstatic on the telephone two weeks earlier. "My tumor markers are coming down," she'd said. "The CEA is down, and the CA 27-29 has dropped from 668 to 420." Her CEA marker had gone down from 90 to 45 in four months. This was good news.

"It looks like the hormones are working," I said, happy for her.

Harriette had thought so, too. We could rest assured that things were stable for now. Today, I was curious to see whether Charlie Blosten's picture was on display in the breast cancer awareness exhibit. He'd mentioned that he had been one of the survivors featured the previous year. Since I'd missed it then, I didn't want to miss it this year if he happened to be featured again as a male survivor.

At the end of the mall I found the glass showcases filled with framed photographs. Some of the cases had five photographs on each side. There were nearly fifty in all. I looked into the eyes of each survivor and read all their names. One was a dancer and another a golfer. There was a tennis player, a mother, and a musician. This disease affected people from all walks of life. But Charlie's picture wasn't among them.

I found more photographs across from the exhibit in the mall's walk-in mammography clinic.

While I was searching for Charlie's photograph, a volunteer asked me whether I wanted a mammogram. "We can help you if you don't have insurance," she said.

"No, I've already had a mammogram, but I was wondering if you have a photograph here of Charlie Blosten? I know his photo was on display here before."

She thought for a moment. "Oh, yes," she said, "I remember him. He gave a speech at the reception at Saks. All the big people with the Komen Foundation and Channel 9 were there." She had just learned a few years before that men could get breast cancer, but she was surprised about Charlie. "He wasn't an old man. He hadn't a mother or a sister with breast cancer. No one in his family had breast cancer. My tears were fallin' so fast, listenin' to him speak."

She looked over all the survivor photographs on the wall. "I guess we don't have Charlie's photo up this year," she said, offering me a calendar and an exhibit
guide on this year's survivor tribute instead. I was disappointed but not with the exhibit she showed me next.

"Have you seen Sarah Hutt's wooden bowls exhibit yet?" she said. "It's called, *My Mother's Legacy*.[1] She led me to several large tables displaying hundreds of brown bowls of every shape and size. "Each bowl says something about her mother, who died from breast cancer when Sarah was just thirteen years old."

She handed me one. I turned the bowl over and read the crude etching on its flat bottom: "My mother kept a dime in her pocket for the phone."[2] I set the bowl back with the others and reached for another: "My mother liked to carry a hanky."[3] Warmth suddenly filled me as I remembered my own mother, who always had a dime and a hanky in her purse. By the third bowl, my breath had escaped me. The sayings were so dear; I wanted to pick up all five hundred bowls. It would have taken a couple of hours to read them all. I read nearly forty, memorizing some of my favorites.

These messages touched me, particularly because they were simple things our mothers said or did that had profound effects in shaping us. It was what made mothers so important and was the reason why we must eradicate breast cancer: to save our mothers.

After I got home, I sat at the kitchen table enjoying the booklets the volunteer had given me. The exhibit guide explained how the idea had come to Sarah Hutt to write her memories on the bottom of the bowls. Her mother, Carmellia Louise Ann Naputano Hutt, "used to turn over pieces of china to see where they'd been made."[4] In the second booklet I discovered to my delight a photograph of Charlie Blosten.

At the quarterly meeting of the Association of Breast Cancer Survivors, I took the seat next to Joyce Coville. Since the first meeting where I met her, I have enjoyed sitting by her. While we waited for the speaker, a physical therapist, to demonstrate some new exercises for combating and preventing lymphedema, Joyce told me her sister had died on September 3rd. "She wanted so badly not to die bald and without breasts, but she died that way anyway." On top of the distress from losing her sister, Joyce was beset by family problems that had suddenly been dropped into her lap as the executor of her sister's estate.

"It sounds like you and I need to go out to lunch," I said. Lately, I'd been feeling rather beset, too. It seemed I always felt like that in September and October, when there was so much going on in my life. When I sensed too many demands on me, I started to crumble, just like I had when I was diagnosed.

I liked Joyce, and I thought lunch together might be therapeutic for both of us.

But she got a pained look on her face. "I can't do it this month. I'm going out of town soon." She had to go to Texas to take care of her sister's affairs.

I was going out of town soon, too, on a much-needed vacation. Although I wanted to be in Denver walking with the sisters in the Race for the Cure on October 6th, I was more excited that Jim and I would be in New Hampshire and Vermont, watching our son Matthew play soccer with his university team.

It was during that vacation that I discovered a swollen lymph node under my arm. It was the arm opposite my mastectomy side, the side I vigilantly checked for lumps and bumps. Although I wasn't particularly worried, I couldn't stop thinking about the little node, nor stop feeling around in my armpit to find it. Sometimes I found it right away, and sometimes I couldn't find it at all. I hated being so paranoid and hated to make a fuss over something if it was nothing, but how could I know if it was or wasn't, if I didn't have it checked? It didn't hurt, but psychologically it annoyed me so much I finally made an appointment with Dr. McAleese. I would have an ultrasound after we got home.

In the examination room, after the technician had finished the ultrasound, I waited for Dr. McAleese. Again, I felt for the swollen node in my armpit. Suddenly, I found something *new* in my breast. It was tiny and hard, like a BB.

When Dr. McAleese came in, she started doing the ultrasound again. "The lymph nodes look totally normal," she said.

"Well, this is really odd, but just now I found something else. What's this?" I had my fingertips pressed into my breast.

She felt the BB too. "I don't know," she said, "but I don't like it. It needs to be biopsied, and I can't do it. You need a surgical biopsy." She wanted me to see Dr. Haun.

My family, Harriette, and Dr. McAleese all seemed worried about the new lump, but Dr. Haun wasn't. "I don't think it's cancer," he said, "but no doctor can tell you for sure, just by how it feels. We can take it out, or we can watch it for a few weeks to see if it gets bigger."

I decided if Dr. Haun wasn't worried about my lump, I wasn't going to worry either. I knew it wouldn't hurt to watch it for a few weeks. Even so, I planned on having him take it out, for Harriette and my family's sake and for my own peace of mind.

The November election was coming up in four days and, over lunch with Harriette, she told me she was going to vote for Tom Strickland for the Senate "because he supports breast cancer research." I nodded and told her I was going in for a breast biopsy.

I could tell it concerned her because she got quiet. Harriette was hardly ever quiet. "I'm not that worried about it," I said. "It's so tiny that even if it *is* cancer, I know I won't need chemotherapy." I didn't tell her I was actually more concerned about the irregular looking, dark black-and-brown mole on my back I'd also decided to have biopsied, along with three others. It seemed too much to put on her now. Those biopsies would occur later anyway.

In the meantime a friend from one of my writing groups called while I was waiting for the pathology results on my breast biopsy. She'd thought to call after she came across information about a publishing workshop she thought I'd be interested in. She talked nervously on the phone. I thought it odd how she was giving me the information so fast and bluntly. I jotted down the particulars even though I had already scheduled two other workshops for the same weekend. I'd been trying to choose between the two of them and now had a third one to consider. "Are you going to this?" I asked.

She paused and then started to cry. "No," she said, "I have breast cancer."

Another woman diagnosed. The numbers of us were increasing. I knew her pain. All of us in the sisterhood knew her pain. We had been in that place. I told her I was a breast cancer survivor. Although she and I had been friends for two years, she hadn't known this before.

My friend was still in shock from receiving the diagnosis two weeks before. Hers was an infiltrating lobular carcinoma, and she was expecting to have bilateral mastectomies and chemotherapy. "I know nothing about my doctors," she said. "They were just recommended by one doctor who knew another doctor who knew another doctor. How do I know if they're good? I just hope I'm making the right decisions."

"I know you have to do this alone," I said, "but you're not in this alone." I cared about her, and I wanted her to know she didn't have to be scared and alone like I had been. There was a whole sisterhood in this with her. She had our support.

Three days after her surgery, as a friend and Reach to Recovery volunteer, I took her some information from the American Cancer Society, along with two temporary breast forms. Later, she wrote me a note, telling me how much that had meant to her.

My breast biopsy report came back as "benign." Dr. Haun said the tissue he removed showed normal fibrocystic changes, just as he had predicted. But, soon again, I was waiting for more biopsy results—on the moles. The one I thought was suspicious, the dermatologist said appeared "more atypical" than the others, so she wanted a more in-depth analysis from a dermatapathologist. The other three moles, she said, were only mildly atypical and were "nothing to worry about."

It seemed ironic to me that most breast cancer survivors fear a recurrence of breast cancer, when the actual killer for me could be a little mole. Malignant melanoma is much deadlier than breast cancer. My first occurrence, in 1987, had been easily excised at an early, curable stage; however, if melanoma is allowed to penetrate deep into the skin, it spreads readily to other organs. Dacarbazine, the drug used for treating advanced melanoma, is one of the most severely toxic chemotherapies of all, and still it's only effective at extending life for a few months.[5]

I would never have to worry about dying from melanoma, I told myself. Although I had a lot of moles, I was vigilant and would be ahead of any that were changing. Nonetheless, I wondered about a correlation between melanoma and breast cancer. *Will I ever, ever get over being paranoid?*

In December it occurred to me that my three-year anniversary as a breast cancer survivor had passed. I felt wonderful. Since Jim was working, I celebrated it privately and cautiously. I was still waiting for results on the one suspicious mole. To fill some time, I looked through our local newspaper, *The High Timber Times,* and was saddened to read in the obituaries that Ernie Krehl, our school bus driver, had died from lung cancer. I remembered Sue Niksic had organized the sock hop to raise money for him, and I imagined she must be upset about his death.

There seemed to be plenty to be concerned about lately: biopsies, moles, deaths, and now tumor markers. Harriette's tumor markers were going up again, slowly. The numbers had come down to 325 but were now over four hundred. We were keeping a vigilant eye on Harriette's markers.

The final report on my suspicious mole had deemed it merely "moderately atypical." What a relief! With a clean bill of health, I decided to pay a visit to Pat Grahn because it'd been a few months since I'd seen her.

I hadn't even mentioned my scare with the little mole yet, when Pat confided that she'd had a scare of recurrence. It turned out to be only a recurrence of paranoia. "In August I had soreness and pain on the right side of my chest where the car seatbelt lay across my neck. I thought my cancer had come back," she said. Pat had just started wearing the car seatbelt again after an admonishment from her primary care doctor. "That's very foolish of you not to use it," he'd scolded when she told him she hadn't been using it since her surgery. It hurt too much.

With that on her conscience, she started wearing it again, and then this pain came. She didn't mention to him or to anyone that she feared the pain was from a recurrence. She just stopped wearing the seatbelt and, eventually, the pain went away. This month she was able to resume wearing the seatbelt without any pain because she'd had the port removed. "The doctor said it was up to me if I felt ready to have it taken out," she said. "I decided to do it."

Pat hadn't realized how uncomfortable the port had been during the past twenty-one months. "On the way home the bumps in the road didn't hurt anymore, and an hour after we'd been home I rubbed my neck, and it felt so good. I feel wonderful again. Now, I only have to try to remember to use the seatbelt," she laughed.

When I next saw Harriette, she shared the highlights of her and Stanley's anniversary trip to Washington, D.C. They'd visited all the national monuments and many museums. They toured the White House, the Capitol, and Congress, spoke with our representative's healthcare aide about the Medicare crisis, and even met with Tom Tancreado himself. For twenty minutes they discussed the issue of prescription drug coverage for seniors.

Harriette, however, had been in considerable pain during the trip. Celebrex and as many as twenty-four Advil tablets a day were no longer working to control the pain radiating from her lower spine. "The Faslodex is not working," she told me while we savored orange peel shrimp at P.F. Chang's. Her tumor markers had been slowly increasing; the CEA had doubled, and the CA-27-29 had jumped from the three hundreds to the four hundreds. It was pointless to get her Faslodex injection this month.

She would have a PET (positron emission tomography) scan after the holidays. PET scans could detect malignant tumors with a high degree of accuracy and could actually measure the living chemistry of the mass. They were more helpful in predicting a patient's outcome.[6] For the scan Harriette would have to have an injection of a radionucleotide combined with sugar that would circulate in her bloodstream and collect in the tumors. The scanning machine would trace the substance and convert it into a visual image on the computer.

"Dr. Jotte said the test would only show them *where* my cancer is, not *how much* there is," Harriette said. He had drawn her a picture describing the cancer. "The cancer is not just one cell. It's hundreds of cells, and sixty percent of them might respond to the medicine by dying while forty percent of them might actually be *feeding* off the hormone. So, stopping the medicine might slow down the growth of those forty percent." Dr. Jotte assured her there were still other options they could try, but first they would have to wait for the PET scan results.

"Cyndi's in a panic about the wait," Harriette said. "She thinks my cancer is going to take off wildly while they're waiting to make decisions about what to try next." In contrast, Harriette wasn't so nervous. She felt cautiously confident that whatever growth was taking place in the tumors would be put in check again with a new treatment. She was just debating whether to buy new clothes at the after-Christmas sales. She wasn't sure she'd be around to wear them.

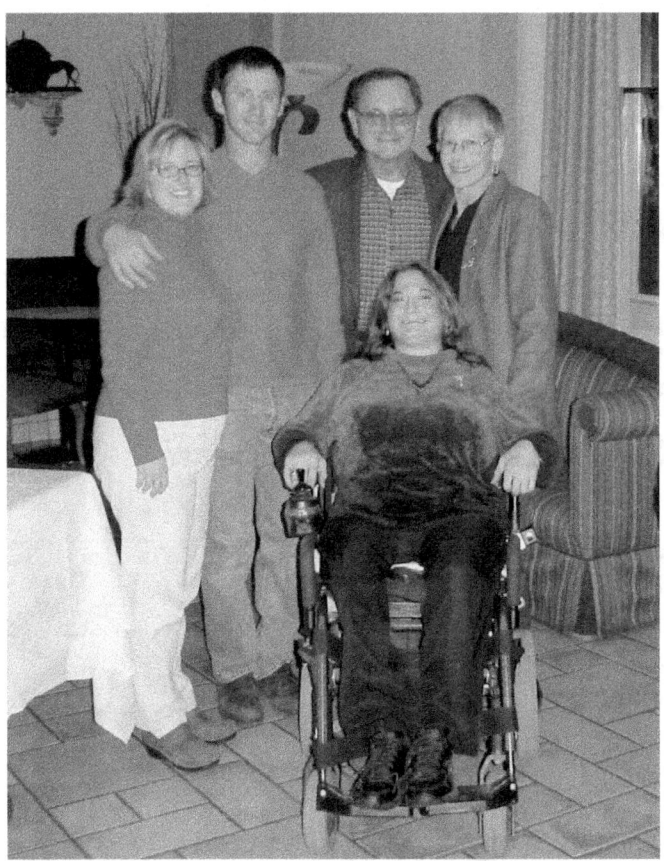

Jill, Jeff, Stanley, Harriette, and Cyndi Grober

CHAPTER 43

Hope and Promise

> "If something happens to her, I will miss my best friend and partner."
>
> Jeff Grober

On New Year's Day the news reported there was plenty of snow at the ski areas. Although it only measured eighty percent of our normal snowfall, I saw it as hope for the drought in Colorado. And the *Today Show* was reporting medical breakthroughs for cancer, "full of hope and promise," that might even come through this year, thanks to twenty-three billion dollars budgeted by Congress. I saw it as hope for Harriette and Sue, whose cancers were not in remission.

As for Harriette, Dr. Jotte was taking her case to the cancer tumor board this week. The tumor board is a group of cancer surgeons, radiation therapists, oncologists, and radiologists, who meet weekly to discuss cases. Since there are no how-to books for oncology, doctors bring their most challenging cases to the board, where all the best and brightest minds can debate treatment options behind closed doors. Each doctor brings opinions based on his or her knowledge and experience. With their pooled expertise, the doctors should ideally leave with the most medically sound treatment plan for their patients.

While the closed doors protect the patients' confidentiality, they also contain the heat that arises sometimes, when the doctors disagree on complex issues. Sometimes they don't agree on a treatment strategy. Harriette's case was indeed complex, but somehow this time they all agreed.

"Dr. Jotte said the board thinks the drug I'm on now is the best way to proceed," Harriette told me. There would be no changes unless her markers were to go up for two consecutive months. Then they would have to try a different hormone. The drug she was taking now was Halotestine, a male hormone. In addition, the doctors concurred, Harriette should see a neurosurgeon for her newly diagnosed spinal stenosis, which they thought was causing her leg and neck pain.

When I heard that Harriette was taking a male hormone, I imagined her needing a "shave" or sounding more like Henry than Harriette, but the only noticeable change was her curly hair. "Did you get a perm?" I asked.

"No," she laughed. "It's called chemotherapy. I've never had curly hair." It had been seven months since she had taken the one treatment of AC and stopped. Harriette was complaining now about having spent twelve hours in the emergency room. Stanley had taken her to the hospital at 3:30 in the morning, when she had awakened in excruciating pain. An MRI had found no tumors, but an orthopedic surgeon had found a new fracture in her pelvic area and displacement of her cervical vertebra. She was still having trouble tipping her head back. "It doesn't hurt when I ride my bike because the handlebars are straight, but I can't read in bed because of my neck pain." After lunch that day, Harriette was going to buy a special pillow for her neck.

The doctor had told her if she fell off her bike and banged her head, she could be paralyzed. "He told me, 'No more riding in the Moonlight Classic. Not because of you,' he said, 'but because of the others. They drink.' It's all right, though," Harriette said. "I had four good years. And they don't serve pancakes at the Moonlight Classic anymore, anyway."

So this is where she'd come. To an acceptance. I'd seen Harriette struggle and fight, yet always she carried on. She never gave up hope. She was an inspiration to me and to others who marveled at her spirit. People speculated on what may have attributed to her longevity with metastatic cancer.

Although she credited it to her exercise and to Aredia, her good friend Anne Weiher told me she thought it was because of how fully Harriette lives her life. "She reaches out and connects with people. She meets and talks with someone every day," Anne said. "She fills up her calendar months in advance, where others live with cancer only day to day, with a goodbye attitude." Anne talked about psychological studies that looked at quality of life. They show that people who are more integrated into society live longer.[1] Anne told me one thing she'd learned from Harriette: "Life can be full and beautiful in the face of imminent death."

Dr. Garfield said that in over thirty years in his profession he couldn't recall anyone else like her. "Harriette is the exception of the exceptions," he said. He couldn't explain her longevity either. "It's something way beyond what we understand. It's more than just mind, body, diet, and exercise."

Harriette was a role model to me, and I wanted to be like her. I wanted to continue on with the groundwork she and others, like Anne Weiher, had laid as advocates with influence on the scientific and medical communities. I wanted to apply to Project LEAD. Maybe I couldn't help Harriette and Sue, but there was something I could do for the sisterhood. I could learn about the science, genetics, and epidemiology of cancer, and I could get trained on how to influence policies that affect breast cancer research and treatment. I wanted to make a difference. Thirty participants from around the country would be selected to participate in one of the science trainings that would be held in Denver during the upcoming year. I applied for one of the slots.

At our next meeting of the ABCS I chose a seat next to Pat Grahn as our new president, a twenty-two-year survivor welcomed us. The topic of discussion that day was a subject of great interest to us: genetic testing. Now that scientists had identified the BRCA1 and BRCA2 genes, many women were considering the pros and cons of having the test done. Some wanted to know whether they were carrying the gene mutations so they could inform their family members to get tested, too. But there was the question of how the information might affect family members and what they would choose to do with it. Some shared the fear that insurance companies might deny coverage if they learned a woman had tested positive for the gene.

One woman, a three-year survivor, said she recently had the test done. "I'd been haunted by the idea that I could be carrying the breast cancer gene even though I've been told I only have a twelve percent chance," she said. Her grandfather had died from breast cancer, and she knew you could get the gene from your father's side. So, she paid nearly $2,800 out-of-pocket for the blood test. The test result was negative, but she said, "It was worth it for my peace of mind." At the conclusion of our discussion, the women were of the opinion that "The test is still controversial."

As I looked around the table, only one person in our group was identifiably undergoing treatment. Her thinned hair was only a half-inch long. As we introduced ourselves, I found out she was Laurel, a three-year survivor of lobular cancer who discovered last August that her cancer had metastasized.

After the meeting, as a group of us stuffed kits for the Reach to Recovery program, I suddenly realized I knew who Laurel was. I had sat next to her at the meeting fifteen months earlier. "I remember you now," I said to her. "I apologize for not recognizing you at first today. You look different without your hair."

"That's all right," she said. "A woman at work said to me, 'You're so bold to get a haircut like that.' I told her I really wasn't bold at all, that this was just nature's way. A bit later Laurel told me privately that the cancer was in her liver now. This was the second time in three years she had lost her hair. The first time had been after her course of AC. "I'm on Taxotere now, and I'm expecting to be on it for the rest of my life," she said in an accepting, matter-of-fact tone. With stage IV cancer, she was hoping to live five more years.

Laurel worked for a large company, tracking data for one of their programs. She was hoping to be able to start doing her job from home soon. "My boss is wonderful," she said. "Sometimes, on my lunch hour I tell him I'm going to take a nap, and I ask him to wake me up in an hour. One day I slept for two and a half hours, and no one said a word to me. My boss just said, 'I figured you needed the rest.' But it would be nice to do my job from home because just getting out of the house in the mornings does me in sometimes."

Besides the fatigue, Laurel said her fingers hurt because fluid had built up behind the nails. The nails were gone now, and she could no longer pick up little things like coins. "I knew the first time I was on chemotherapy that my cancer could come back, so I've been vigilant with follow-up ever since. My doctors and I were on top of this recurrence right away." Laurel said she wasn't worried much about what was to come. "I figure when it's your time, it's your time."

My heart went out to her. Any of us could be in her shoes. As the ladies prepared to leave, Pat Grahn pulled me aside and told me she wanted to tell me about her recent follow-up appointment with her doctor. I hoped she didn't have bad news. "I've been feeling so good lately that I said to my doctor, 'I have all of my energy back now, and I'm doing fine, so I really don't think I need to come in every three months anymore.'" Pat said she'd felt embarrassed that perhaps she'd gotten a little too cocky because then he had gotten very serious and said, "Yes. You do need to come in every three months. It's very important."

My eyes welled up when Pat said that. "I'm happy you're feeling so great, and it's good your doctor cares enough to be so watchful." At the same time, the fact that her cancer was still a threat tugged at my heart.

When I read the headline "Why?" in the *Rocky Mountain News* on February 3rd, I immediately thought of the question: Why are we getting breast cancer? But the headline wasn't asking that. Just because a lot of *my* world seemed to revolve around cancer didn't mean the rest of the world was so obsessed.

The headline was referring to the flashing lights that had streamed over the Texas sky early Saturday morning. The question was, Why had the space shuttle Columbia suddenly disintegrated right before our eyes? It had happened fifteen minutes before it was scheduled to land in Florida. In an instant the world lost seven extraordinary people and a space shuttle full of valuable scientific information, including one experiment related to cancer. It left heaviness in our hearts that still lingered the day after the disaster, as Jim and I drove Matthew to the airport. Behind his quiet reserve, I could tell Matthew was ecstatic. Twenty-one years old now, he was going to Brisbane, Australia, to study for a semester. Over the last three weeks I'd watched him devour several books about the country.

In spite of our somber mood, there was no lingering at the passenger drop-off. We had time for only a few words and a hug. "Thank you, so much, Mom and Dad, for letting me do this," he said.

"I love you," I said, holding him tightly, and then he turned and walked away. We watched him disappear into the terminal with all of his belongings stuffed into his backpack and one small travel case. He didn't see our tears as we drove away.

Jim and I were too emotional to speak for a while. Our son had traveled around the United States with his competitive soccer teams since he was twelve years old, but this was the first time I'd seen him truly excited about going somewhere new. I imagined that fifteen days before Houston lost contact with the space shuttle, the parents of those astronauts had felt like I did today—proud and happy, sad, nervous, and scared, yet resigned to "letting go." We have to let our children follow their passions and do what they love. They're hopeful about the future, and when they're happy, they make a difference in the world. As my kids had grown up, they'd seen Jim and I follow our passions, and now we were watching them follow theirs.

I was looking for things to feel good and positive about. Our country was on the verge of war against Iraq. We'd just had another shuttle disaster, and, right after it, I had put my youngest child on an airplane that was taking him halfway around the world. With so much uncertainty in the world, I felt it possible I might never see him again. I was uneasy, too, about what might happen to Harriette and the fact that we still didn't know the cause of breast cancer.

Kim Scott, my young survivor friend, believed as I did that stress had caused our immune systems to go haywire. But since my diagnosis in 1999, I had read no studies that pointed to this as a single cause. I found one study, published in the October 2002 *Journal of the National Cancer Institute*, that squelched the idea that antiperspirants cause cancer.[2] Researchers in Washington State found no correlation between breast cancer and the use of either deodorants or antiperspirants after underarm shaving with razor blades. The theory of an environmental cause, however, strongly remained.

Although Harriette and I had never discussed it, I recalled the early 90s, when residents of the area of Long Island, where she was from, became loudly vocal about their concern over the high incidence of breast cancer cases in their region. Even though Harriette was no longer a Long Island resident, I imagined at the time she'd been very attentive to this issue.

I decided to look up the study and found out the Long Island Breast Cancer Study Project had come about in 1993, after it was discovered that approximately two thousand cases of in situ and invasive breast cancer were being diagnosed annually in Nassau and Suffolk counties.[3] The realization roused a group of grassroots activists in New York to begin pressuring Congress to mandate a study into the matter. When Congress authorized the study, it was mandated to be completed as soon as possible.

So, an elaborate $30 million project was funded by the National Cancer Institute and the National Institute of Environmental Health Sciences, to look at what environmental pollutants these women might have been exposed to in the drinking water and the air. Additionally, researchers performed electromagnetic field studies to assess the influence on melatonin levels, which affect estrogen levels, and they tested the soil for residues of organochlorine compounds, which were formerly used in pesticides and in electrical equipment. Although the compounds had been banned for years prior to the study, they are believed to be stored in fatty tissue and to act as hormones do in the body.

The project studied residents recently diagnosed with breast cancer and a control group of women who did not have breast cancer. However elaborate, the study was limited. It was unable to assess what the women may have been exposed to decades earlier.

When I shared with Harriette what I had learned about this study, she said she'd been too occupied with her cancer treatment during that time to be able to pay much attention to it. But she did remember once talking to a woman involved with the research. It was when Harriette had been in New York visiting her mother. "Other than that, I wasn't involved, but I do remember the trucks that sprayed DDT to kill the mosquitoes. As kids we ran after the trucks near the Yankee Stadium in the Bronx. All the kids did that."

Harriette wasn't familiar with any of the specifics of the study. "What was the outcome?" she wanted to know.

"They found no link between the pollutants and breast cancer," I said. The researchers had found low levels of the organochlorine compounds in *both* groups and determined, therefore, that the organochlorines were unassociated with breast cancer. The researchers weren't able to rule out the possibility that earlier exposure to higher levels of organochlorines might have caused an increased risk of breast cancer.[4]

The study left room for me to believe that environmental toxicity could be a cause for breast cancer, but as Barron Lerner, M.D., author of *The Breast Cancer Wars*, said in a journal article: "Studies that attempt to identify carcinogenic substances are notoriously difficult to do. Activists and researchers may need to acknowledge that a link between breast cancer and environmental toxins, if it exists, may be impossible to prove."

If cancer is caused by genetic mutations, I thought, then these were hereditary and had nothing to do with an impaired immune system. Didn't dinosaurs have cancer, too? But if cancer *is* caused by environmental pollutants, then we have a very long way to go in identifying them and cleaning them up to prevent cancer in the future.

As I read more, I learned that much of the research on cancer is focused on genes and is leading to proteins onto which therapies may be specifically targeted. These so-called molecular targets may radically change the course of breast cancer treatment in the future. As Gwen Darien, former editor-in-chief of *MAMM* magazine, said in the February 2003 issue, the research in the last five years has switched from "detect and destroy" to "target and control." It appears that, instead of eradicating cancer, science is making incremental improvements in learning how to live with it. But for women like Harriette, Sue, and Laurel, who didn't have much time to wait for the cure, it seemed like research was moving at a snail's pace. One thing slowing research, according to Gwen Darien, was that fewer than five percent of cancer patients participate in clinical trials. They just don't want to be guinea pigs.

I began to understand what other obstacles were slowing research down, most of them related in one way or another to the need for money. Funds were needed to pay for things like: increased research on the biology and developmental genetics of the normal mammary gland, research on the genetics and biology of precancerous lesions and their progression to invasive, metastatic cancers, and funding for new technologies and equipment.[5] Other needs were strategies for researchers to be able to share access to resources such as the microarray/chip technology and ways for academia and industry to form partnerships on new drug development.

As we were soon to engage in war with Iraq, which we hoped to win, I hoped for Harriette, Sue, and Laurel's sakes that, by addressing these research obstacles, scientists would soon be winning the war on cancer.

CHAPTER 44

Sixty Miles toward Conquering Breast Cancer

Just as Harriette and Charlie Blosten had become involved with advocacy for breast cancer and I had applied for Project LEAD, Kim Scott had gotten involved in her own way. She wanted to help scientists win the war on cancer, so she joined the Avon Breast Cancer Crusade. I knew she had recently participated in the Avon 3-Day in California, and when I called to congratulate her on completing the walk, she told me some other exciting news. "I got engaged," she said.

She and her boyfriend had been together for two years, and now they were planning a wedding. I met her a few weeks later for lunch at Cucina Colore and marveled over her new marquis diamond ring, happy to see a young woman getting on with her future after breast cancer. I was most eager, too, to hear about her walk to Malibu. In my mind I saw her in bare feet at the water's edge, holding her worn-out tennis shoes, looking out onto the bright future on the horizon. A future without breast cancer. It was the perfect ending to her walk.

Kim and her friend Sarah had walked for three days on a sixty-mile mission to raise funds to pay for early detection for the underserved and for breast cancer research. I'd never participated in one of the walks. "What was the 3-Day like?" I asked.

"It was Sarah's idea to do the walk in California," Kim said. "She wanted to get involved in one of the thirteen Avon walks that were going on nationwide. Since she had gone to school in Santa Barbara, she wanted to do the walk there. She asked me to do it with her."

Their Santa Barbara walk was to begin on October 18th, following the opening ceremonies at the Earl Warren Show Grounds. The route meandered for sixty miles through neighborhoods, along highways, and down the Pacific Coast, with one overnight camp on Ventura State Beach. The walk would culminate in a closing ceremony on Zuma Beach at Malibu on October 20th. But first, Kim and Sarah had to spend time training and getting in shape.

"We started our training in June," Kim said, "slacking a bit at first. We walked only once a week in Washington Park for a couple of hours, and then I stopped altogether for the month of July because I moved. We picked up again in September, when we started walking with Sarah's dogs, Max and Bogie."

They were walking twice around the park, five or six miles, two times a week. By October they had worked up to twelve miles each time.

Shoes were the biggest problem for Kim during the training. "I tried several pairs, and every one bothered my feet. They didn't work well for walking long distances. Then a woman at a sporting women's store in Cherry Creek finally helped me find the right shoes for my feet. She watched me walk in them and even let me march around the block once, to try them out." Ultimately, Kim settled on a pair of Asics—just in time for the event. Kim and Sarah were physically strong. They were ready.

Five days before they were to check in for the Avon walk, where they would be constantly on foot, sweating, hurting, and sleeping in tents, Kim and Sarah flew out to Santa Barbara. "We wanted to pamper ourselves for a few days first, so we checked into the Biltmore Hotel, looked around the town, shopped, had pedicures, and generally enjoyed ourselves."

On Thursday the 18th the two young survivors arrived at the welcome center, where 4,443 walkers, including 420 survivors, were gathering for registration. The registration process seemed to take forever. But there was growing excitement, with people coming from all over for the cause. With each one required to raise a minimum of $1,900 for the entry, the pledges already totaled over $6 million. Kim and Sarah watched safety videos and enjoyed the food while they waded through the process and observed all the people.

At registration everyone was surprised to be informed there had been a change in the route because of the large number of walkers. The ending point was no longer going to be at Malibu Beach. The Zuma Beach area, originally planned for the closing ceremony, would not be able to accommodate all the people. Instead, at the end of each day of walking, the walkers would be bussed to a camp surrounded by trees at a university campus in Oxnard, where two thousand blue tents were set up. The end of the walk and the closing ceremony would be held there, at Oxnard.

Early the next morning, while it was still dark, the two dressed in shorts, tank tops, and running shoes and filled their camel backs with one hundred ounces of water. With sunscreen, sandals, and cameras stuffed into daypacks, they strolled onto the fairgrounds carrying nearly fifteen pounds on their backs, with the rest of their gear in duffel bags. "I wanted to be comfortable," Kim said, "so before we went out to California, I invested in the camel back, a good Therma Rest pad made of half foam and half air, and a good sleeping bag. All of my equipment together only weighed thirty-five pounds." Her equipment would prove to be a good investment.

After picking up their route maps and leaving their sleeping gear at the drop-off point, Kim and Sarah joined the throng crowding toward the opening ceremony. There were walkers of every age, from seventeen to seventy-seven. Walkers and teams with names like "Mommies on a Mission" and "Hookers for Hooters" were all bunched together. "Team TaTa" wore pink hats and carried pink balloons. "We had long fluorescent pink wigs that we were saving to wear on the last day," Kim said.

In the stadium, tremendous energy emanated from the crowd, united behind one cause. "It was incredibly inspirational," Kim said. "The opening prayers and speeches brought back all that each of us had been through, and there was so much emotion, everyone had tears streaming down their faces." The cool breeze of the morning boosted her adrenalin, and on that high Kim and Sarah started their walk.

They trekked through the city of Santa Barbara and along the coastline, heading to the Bluffs at Carpinteria. "After only five miles, I was so tired I thought, my God how am I going to walk sixty miles? But people were cheering us on and handing out bananas, oranges, and peanut butter snacks at every pit stop, so we kept on." At the end of the first day, they had logged seventeen miles.

"The second day was the hardest for me, though not as difficult as I expected it to be, because after walking seventeen miles, it was like my body had assimilated to the walking, and I was ready for another day." The route took them past Channel Islands Harbor, where the light sea breeze kept them from getting hot as they traipsed on through the Mandalay Beach community. In the afternoon they trudged along a boardwalk above the beach and onto the Main Street of Ventura.

"We saw dolphins and some beautiful scenery along the way, but a lot of places weren't so pretty. We had to walk through stickers and straw, and there was no place to sit except on the dirt." Toward the end of the day they were so tired that Kim could hardly remember where they had walked, but there was one span of five miles along Harbor Boulevard where there was so much traffic they'd had to walk in single file. "We were all talked out by then anyway, so it wasn't so bad." It was just a matter of putting one foot in front of the other.

After eighteen miles, their second day of walking came to an end at a bus stop. "It should have felt great being finished for the day, but we had to stand in line for another hour with hundreds of other walkers while we waited for the buses. When they finally came, we were so grateful to be able to sit down." They were the nicest buses Kim had ever seen. She and Sarah sank into the soft seats—two tired, dirty souls—and relished the twenty-minute ride back to camp.

"The Avon 3-Day was not a great experience because of what we were seeing," Kim said. "It was great because of what we were doing. We were on a serious mission. We were there to walk." During the days they didn't talk much about anything except where they could expect to find the next set of port-a-potties and what they were going to do when they got their shoes off. "Sometimes, we didn't talk at all. Mostly, we were obsessed with avoiding blisters." When they stopped to rest or took off their socks at the end of the day, they saw holes had worn right through the blister patches. Because of that, they nearly panicked when they started running out of them. Once they even went into Rite Aid and, at $5 a pack, bought all they had. "In all, we spent nearly $100 on those patches. They became the most important thing in our lives during those three days."

"Weren't you exhausted at night from all that walking?" I asked.

"Oh, my god, yes. But they fed us well, and the hot showers at the end were the most wonderful." Kim never expected that a shower on a truck could feel so good. "They had events going on at night. We could hear people enjoying them, but after we ate the spaghetti and cheesecake served by the volunteers, Sarah and I went to our tent." So they could find theirs easily in the sea of blue, they had decorated their tent on the outside with pink pig puppets they got from a hair salon. They took off their shoes before they climbed in. "We slept wonderfully."

The third day, the duo filled their camel backs with water for the last time and donned their long, neon pink wigs, complete with bangs and sunglasses, for the final fourteen miles. All day they trudged, wearing their wigs through the city of Oxnard and onto Rose Avenue before hitting the home stretch. "We had tasted every flavor of Gatorade at rest stops throughout those three days. By the last day, I'd had enough Gatorade to last me a lifetime."

During the last few miles Kim was walking on so much adrenalin she could have gone another twenty miles—even with her blisters. "Our wigs had been such a hit, Sarah and I wish now we had worn them the whole time."

A huge band of screaming, cheering people, half a mile long, welcomed them at the end, where all the survivors got pink T-shirts and the other walkers got blue. At the closing speeches, they sat in rows of blue on the outside and pink on the inside. In the innermost row were the volunteers. As they listened to the speakers, both Kim and Sarah cried. They had walked in the very last Avon 3-Day by Pallotta Teamworks. The first had begun in Santa Barbara in 1998. Altogether, the walks had raised more than $116 million. "It was the most wonderful experience of my life," Kim said. "It was a mental thing, a strife that paralleled conquering breast cancer. We did it to help the underprivileged and to aid research. We survived breast cancer, and walking sixty miles was the proof."

CHAPTER 45

Blizzard and War

Maybe it was the coming of spring that made me ready for change, but in March I finally opened up to Dr. Huang's suggestion and allowed her to do a "lift" on my right breast. She'd been offering me that option since she did the original reconstruction of my left breast. Mine hadn't matched since the reconstruction because the implanted breast was firm and round, and the natural one was supple and tear-dropped. I'd been reluctant to have a lift because I thought my breast was fine the way it was. But she convinced me that with time and age the lopsided discrepancy would become more apparent. My implanted breast was a little too firm anyway. It had no "give," and I'd not been able to sleep on my stomach for three years. Dr. Huang would remove the implant and replace it with a smaller, "softer" one and do the "lift" on the other breast. I was psychologically ready for the change.

Afterward, though black-and-blue, swollen, and sore, I was immediately pleased with the results. I was still recovering when the snow came. It had been falling steadily for over an hour as Jim and I sat at the kitchen table listening to President Bush address the world on national television: "Saddam Hussein and his sons must leave Iraq within forty-eight hours. Their refusal to do so will result in military conflict commenced at a time of our choosing," he said. It seemed the United States was ready for change, too—a regime change in Iraq. For twelve years Saddam Hussein had been in violation of the disarmament agreement. Now, President Bush warned that a coalition was going to "enforce the just demands of the world."

A short time after the president said his ominous goodnight, I noticed Jim outside in his shirtsleeves. He was fiddling with something under the hood of our old Chevy truck while the snow flew around him. As he often did with the plow truck, he was having problems again, and the battery was brand new. I had bought it just a week earlier. The problem had to be an electrical one. I thought we were in for it. A blizzard was forecast with an accumulation of six feet expected. We'd be stuck without the plow working. Inside the house I shivered with worry over what was coming—a blizzard and a war.

Eventually, I saw Jim had the truck running. From our living room window I watched him coming down our long driveway, the plow pushing the snow out to the sides and in front of the truck. Adept and sure from years of experience, he moved at a steady clip, stopping just short of the retaining wall where the driveway ended in a twelve-foot drop-off. The plow pushed the snow over the wall. At the same speed he backed up the driveway and came down again in another pass.

For years I'd watched Jim plow from our windows that look out into the forest, and still I took a breath each time he came to the end at the retaining wall, praying he'd stop before his front wheels dipped over the edge. He always stopped at the right second. That night, he made another pass and another, until the driveway was cleared down to a snow pack, and we went to bed.

By early morning, there were four feet of snow on the deck and more than three feet covered the length of the driveway. Jim started the plow truck again. He thought he would clear the driveway so we could get out and go to work, but it was soon evident that we weren't going anywhere. During the night the county snowplow had made one swipe on the road past our house and blocked us in. Jim would have to hand-shovel the top of the driveway, chain up the plow truck, and work backward up the driveway.

I called to cancel my interpreting assignment. Instead of going to work, I dressed in snow pants and Sorrels and, in spite of my recent surgery, took a shovel to the deck. We wanted the weight of the snow off to avoid the risk of it collapsing. In place of lifting the snow over the rails, I pushed shovelfuls through the openings under them. The snow dropped into the piles below, landing with a soft thud. The ground was normally fourteen feet below our deck, but as the snow piled higher, it was reaching toward the deck. Beneath me, the snow heaped past the top of the sliding glass door and past the windows in our basement. Soon, we could no longer see out from them. We felt buried.

The snow fell steadily all day. We'd never seen so much snow! Another foot accumulated, and Jim had to plow again. He moved the truck silently up and down the driveway. The high drifts insulated all sound. Before long there was no place left to push any more snow. Jim's plowing had formed a snow wall ten feet high, and the clean circle in front of the house was getting smaller and smaller. Our driveway, big enough for six cars, had barely room for two.

The next morning there were close to seven feet in the middle of the deck, where we hadn't removed any snow the day before. The county snowplows still hadn't cleared the main road, and we were truly snowbound. It snowed all day, and more inches accumulated. Even the elk were looking for plowed roads on which to walk. From the deck I watched a bull moving slowly through the drifts, lifting his hooves high. The snow came up past his belly. Stuck at home on the first day of spring, I canceled my follow-up appointment with Dr. Huang and my sign language lesson with Bert. People were complaining of cabin fever, but I loved being snowbound. It allowed me time to read.

The news reported the snow pack had reached 110 percent of normal in some areas. We had received some good medicine for our drought. After four years of too little precipitation, this blizzard was still not enough to refill our shrunken mountain reservoirs, but, come spring, it would raise water levels considerably.

On Saturday the sun shone over our glistening white wonderland, and we were finally out on the road. We could see what had walloped Colorado. People everywhere were experiencing the side

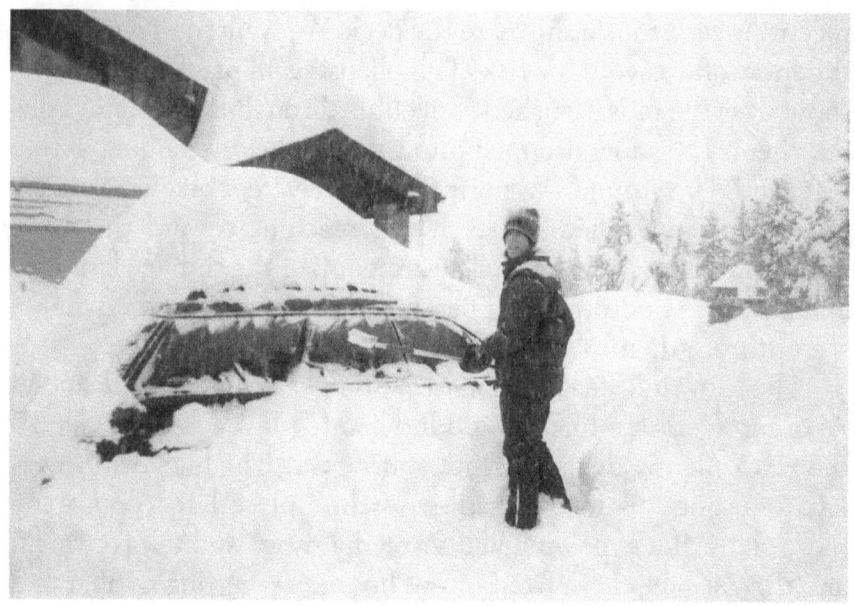

Me, shoveling out from our seven-foot blizzard.

effects of this medicine. Like little termites, those near us, who weren't able to plow their driveways, were starting to poke their heads out of tunnels they'd dug from their homes to the main road. Everyone was talking about how to get heavy commercial equipment to move the wet tons of white. Snowplows and snow blowers were practically useless. The snow was too heavy.

For those of us who had dug out early, driving on the mountain was treacherous. It was slippery and slushy, walking or driving. I found the trick was to drive fast enough so I didn't get stuck if I stopped, but then the slush pulled my car where it wanted and made for a turbulent ride. I didn't want to go too fast either, for fear of suddenly meeting another car head-on in only one lane.

In the town of Conifer, the snowplows had cleared narrow passages where walls of snow eight to ten feet high paneled each side. Like driving through a maze, I had no idea where the next turn was or what would be around its corner. The snow took up space everywhere. The grocery store was open, but parking was at a premium. Some parked their trucks on top of the snow mounds.

I gave up on stopping at the grocery store and kept moving, only to compete again for the scant parking at the post office. After five days we mountain residents were clamoring to pick up our undelivered mail.

We hadn't seen a newspaper in five days either, but we knew from television that bombs had been dropping on Baghdad. We were fortunate to have had electrical power for the news to keep us informed during the storm. Many others hadn't. What we didn't know was whether Saddam Hussein was alive or dead. It was thought the first "surgical strike" onto his palace might have wounded or killed him. Nevertheless, the precision-guided missiles continued firing on Iraq's military targets, exactly where they were supposed to, and not onto Iraqi civilians. It was more humanitarian to spare the innocent and the healthy parts of Iraq while we tried to rid the world from this oppressive and brutal regime.

Scientists use the same theory in the war on cancer. To develop and use less disfiguring, invasive, and toxic treatments, they're zeroing in on the malignancy and aiming to spare healthy cells. As their studies on the molecular level advance, they're making strides on this track. They're identifying cancer proteins onto which we hope to aim treatments more specifically, and they're studying gene activity to learn which tumors are more likely to spread and which may need more aggressive treatments. We have hope that by fixing mutated genes scientists might someday be able to alter the defects that allow cells to transform into cancer.

While we were snowbound, I immersed myself in reading about cancer. I read about the progress scientists are making. I found it fascinating, exciting, and hopeful. New techniques in cancer treatment are entering the trial stages, including immunotherapy, which uses altered cells from the tumor itself in such a way that they may stimulate an immune response against the cancer, and vaccines, which might someday be able to customize our treatment to the specific characteristics of our tumors. Scientists are also looking to the sea now, which may hold the secret to cancer treatment. They already have clinical trials underway for sea squirt toxin, an agent they say is one hundred times more powerful than Taxol.[1]

The aromatase inhibitors are in clinical trials and are working well to prevent estrogen from stimulating cancer cell growth.

As I read, I learned how cancer develops. Simply, it develops from damaged DNA in a cell. There are many combining factors that contribute to damaged DNA or damage to our genes. I'd learned about most of these contributing factors in college: stress, diet, too little exercise, obesity, environmental toxins, and a predisposition governed by what genes we have inherited. What I hadn't heard of before was the factor of excess estrogen. How might someone have too much estrogen?

According to Dr. John R. Lee (*What Your Doctor May Not Tell You About Breast Cancer*), things in our environment, like pesticides, solvents, plastics, carpet, furniture, and even nail polish, give off chemicals that act like estrogen in the body. He says that when the body can't break the chemicals down properly, we have an imbalance that wreaks havoc on our cells. If our own natural repair mechanisms can't get rid of the estrogen, it causes mutations in genes. The mutations don't always cause cancer, but sometimes they do.

Since I've never been overweight and environmental toxins and a predisposition seemed like things I had no control over, I didn't concern myself with them. I'd never thought about things like electromagnetic fields and nail polish giving me cancer. I'd long ago stopped insisting my family eat brown rice instead of instant rice, and I had stopped worrying about whether they ate their broccoli and cauliflower. But now, I was reconsidering these things.

My daughter Heather loves to wear nail polish. I would hate to think that her innocent use of it could give her breast cancer. Separately, I doubted it would, but together with car exhaust, new carpet fumes, paint, and other toxins she might absorb through her skin, as well as using birth control pills, eating poorly, or not exercising enough, perhaps nail polish could be one more contributing factor. To my knowledge there is no scientific evidence linking nail polish to breast cancer. It was something to think about.

It's unlikely that we will ever eliminate all of the factors that contribute to cancer. Nevertheless, Dr. Lee's book reminded me about things I could do for myself and for my family to decrease our risk. such as: stop microwaving food in plastic wrap to prevent the di-(2-ethylhexyl)adipate from seeping into the food and stop standing in front of the microwave while it's cooking.

I resolved to reduce the sugar from our diet and to serve more broccoli and cauliflower so we might benefit from their indole-3-carbinol properties. And I would impart information to my daughter so she will have a better opportunity to prevent breast cancer in herself. With our individual diligence and the advancements in research, I believe my daughter and future granddaughters will not have to deal with mastectomies and reconstruction.

As good things sometimes emerge from bad, after our snowstorm subsided I saw people starting to emerge from shelter. I saw neighbors I don't normally see, and I talked to Sue Niksic. I called her to see how her family was faring and to invite her to go to the Day of Caring, which was coming up again in May. "We're still buried," she said. "I need to get out, so I can get my chemotherapy on Thursday." Her husband had left their jeep on the road, she said, so he was able to go to work, but she was home with the kids.

That she was on chemotherapy was news to me. The last time we had spoken, Sue was on Arimidex, and her cancer had been stabilized. The fact that the hormones had stopped working was not good news.

Last fall when she began losing weight and having abdominal bloating, she suspected her cancer was active again. "The doctors thought it was something wrong with my gall bladder since my markers were only up slightly."

They removed her gall bladder, but the bloating only became worse, to the point that she couldn't eat or hardly drink, and she ended up in the hospital, twice. "I had so much fluid built up, I couldn't walk, because I couldn't bend my toes," Sue said. I've never felt that awful before. I honestly didn't think I was going to make it." It was the first time since her diagnosis that she'd thought that. The doctor put her on a diuretic while she was hospitalized, and she lost thirty-seven pounds of excess fluid in ten days.

"My kids know about my cancer now. I told them in January, when I went into the hospital. But they already knew. My eleven-year-old son asked me if I was going to die. I said, 'Maybe I won't live as long as most people, but I'm doing okay now.'"

I could tell in her voice and by the fact that her kids knew that she had come to an acceptance. Nevertheless, Sue sounded upbeat in spite of the recent turn in events and the fact that she had lost her hair again, for the third time. "My liver is much better now. I can eat again." Her only complaints were from the side effects of Taxotere. "I ache all over, and the skin on my hands and feet peels."

I felt bad that I hadn't known she was sick again. Sue admitted she didn't like telling people about her cancer. "I don't mind talking about it after they know I have it, but I just can't tell them."

I knew what she meant. I had been that way, too. But now I had the sisterhood in my life, and it gave me a strength I never had before. We brought strength to each other, and I hoped that in some small way I could bring some to Sue. I told her I wanted her to meet the other women who had also become my friends during this journey into the world of breast cancer: Kim, Sarah, Pat, and Harriette.

I was deeply concerned about Sue, as I was for Harriette, but Harriette's markers were going down now on the hormone, Halotestin. There was still hope. There was always hope. I told Sue I would request a scholarship for her registration to the Day of Caring, and she said she'd like that.

When May came, however, and it was time for the Day of Caring, I was disappointed because Sue was too sick and weak to go. I went by myself.

Sorting through the letters from the mailbox, I found one addressed to me. I stepped down our driveway, reading the letter, which informed me I'd been accepted for Project LEAD. I would be able to become an informed advocate for breast cancer. I could carry on Harriette's work. At that joyful moment I became aware of the familiar sound coming from our stream. It was the rippling rush we hadn't heard the year before. Thanks to the blizzard, there was water in our stream again. Perhaps our drought was over. The rejuvenating sound with the letter in hand gave me hope, for myself and for the sisterhood.

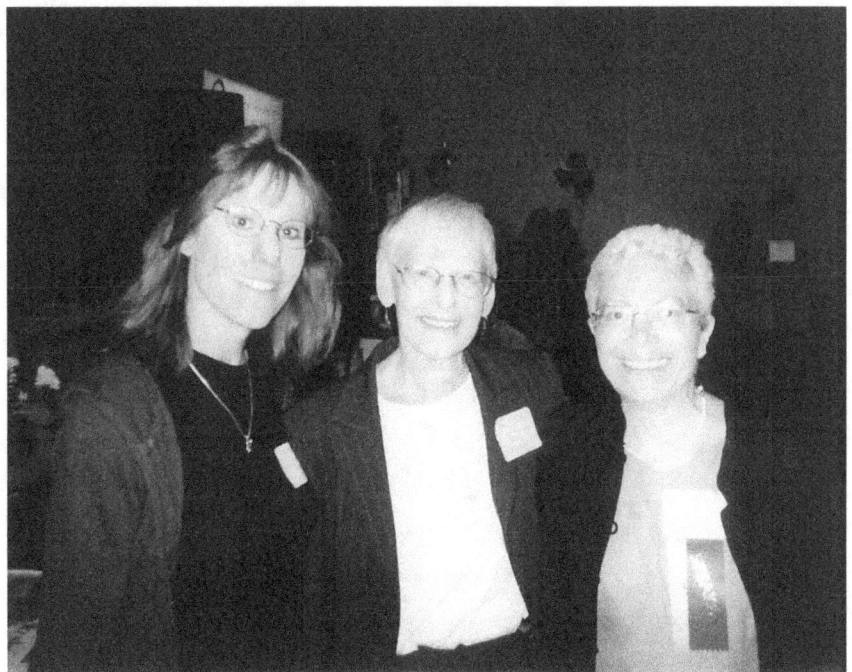

Diane, Harriette, and Vicki Tosher at the Day of Caring, May 2004.

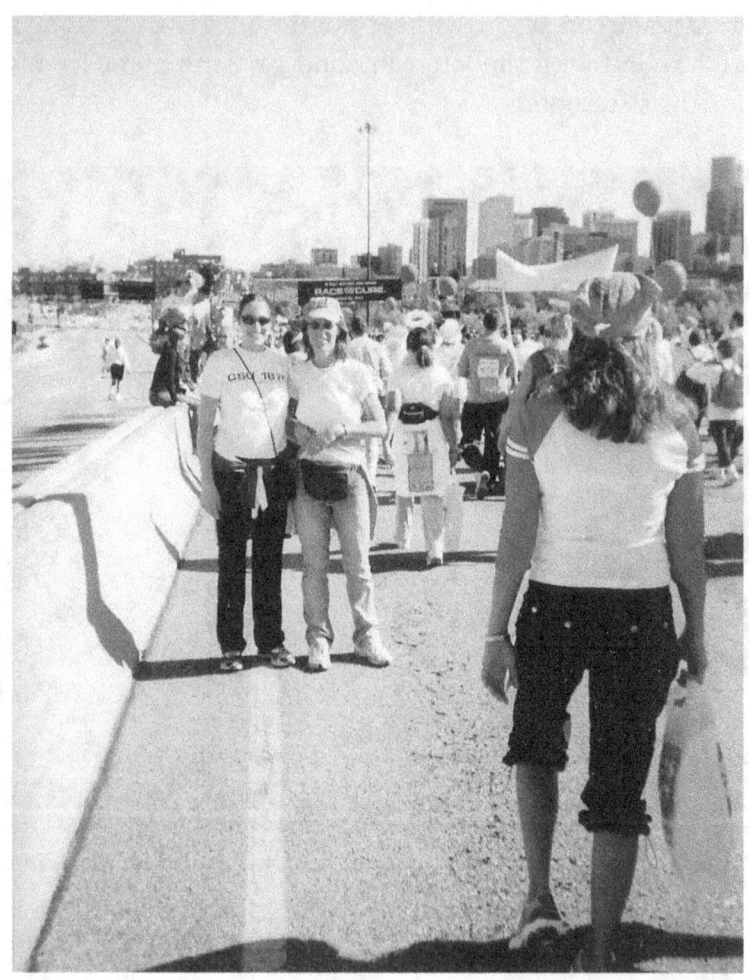
Heather and me at Race for the Cure in Denver, October 2004.

EPILOGUE

At the end of the summer in 2004, my daughter and I signed up to participate in the Race for the Cure. We planned to meet Harriette and Cyndi at the starting line of the one-mile family walk near the Pepsi Center in downtown Denver. Sensing that this race could be Harriette's last, it was especially important to us.

On October 3rd, the day of the race, we arrived to find what I heard reported later were 63,458 walkers—a record number for any Race for the Cure anywhere. People were already flowing over the starting line and streaming along the viaduct, where normally there were motor vehicles. With Harriette and Cyndi nowhere in sight, my daughter, her roommate, and I stepped in with the flow. For the next several hours the three of us walked in the sunshine amid a peaceful, orderly crowd. Survivors like me wore pink T-shirts and pink visors. Pinned to the back of my shirt I wore a sign: "I Race In Memory of Sue Niksic."

A few weeks after the race I grew worried when I hadn't been able to reach Harriette for a couple of days. She'd found out recently and informed me that the cancer in her lungs was worse and had spread to her liver. I was relieved when she finally called on a Sunday afternoon. "I'm in the hospital," she said. She told me she was having trouble breathing.

"Can I come see you?" I asked.

"You better," she said. "You're my sister. I never had a sister before." She told me she would be in the hospital for a couple of days.

The next day when I arrived at the hospital, Harriette was in bed wearing a hospital gown and the bicycle charm necklace I had given her for her birthday. Her family and lots of visitors were there. More people came throughout the day, into the evening, and for several more days after she was moved into hospice. There were many friends, some whom I knew and others she'd mentioned to me. I was not surprised to learn of the others. As I spoke to many, I learned that Harriette had telephoned each one to let them know she was "crossing over to the other side."

In Memory of
Sue Niksic, March 2, 1959–March 10, 2004
and
Harriette Grober, March 28, 1942–October 26, 2004

NOTES

CHAPTER 3
1. Boys Town National Research Hospital, National Center for the Study and Treatment of Usher Syndrome, www.boystownhospital.org/UsherSyndrome/index.asp, accessed February 2004.
2. Susan M. Love, with Karen Lindsey, *Dr. Susan Love's Breast Book*, third edition (Cambridge: Perseus Publishing, 2000), 61–62.

CHAPTER 9
1. Ellen Leopold, *A Darker Ribbon: A Twentieth-Century Story of Breast Cancer, Women, and Their Doctors* (Boston: Beacon Press, 1999), 23.

CHAPTER 11
1. *Dr. Susan Love's Breast Book*, 490.

CHAPTER 12
1. Ibid., 383.

CHAPTER 23
1. Cynthia O'Dell, "Meet DePauw's New Faculty Members," *DePauw Magazine*, "Artist and Activist, Feature Section" (Fall 1998), 21.

CHAPTER 24
1. Amy D'Orazio and Kavita Maung, "Drug Therapies," *CURE* 1.4 (December 2002): 70.

CHAPTER 25
1. Beth Murphy, *Fighting for Our Future: How Young Women Find Strength, Hope, and Courage While Taking Control of Breast Cancer* (New York: McGraw Hill, 2003), 10.

CHAPTER 26
1. Kathy LaTour, "Lost in the Fog: Breast Cancer and Chemobrain," *CURE* 1.1 (Premier Issue, 2002): http://www.curetoday.com/backissues/v1n1/features/chemobrain/index.html, accessed 5 May 2006.

CHAPTER 27
1. *Zometa, Prescribing Information* (Novartis Oncology, March 2002).

CHAPTER 40
1. Alice McCarthy, "Combining the Old & New against colon cancer," *CURE* 1.4 (December 2002): 34.

CHAPTER 42
1. Sarah Hutt, *My Mother's Legacy*, www.mymotherslegacy.com, accessed 2006.
2. Ibid.
3. Ibid.
4. Centura Health, *Exhibit Guide*, "We Speak to Honor, A Photographic Celebration of Survival at Cherry Creek Shopping Center," 2002.
5. Ralph W. Moss, *Questioning Chemotherapy* (Brooklyn, NY: Equinox Press, 1995), 131–132.
6. Dr. Koop, "Pet Scans Give Breast Cancer Victims Peace of Mind," http://www.drkoop.com/template.asp?page=newsdetail&ap=93&id=506242, 2-4-03.

CHAPTER 43
1. Deborah Mitchell and Deborah Gordon, *Breast Health the Natural Way* (New York: John Wiley and Sons, 2001), 136. Dr. David Spiegel's ten-year study tracking the progress of women with metastasized breast cancer.
2. Dana K. Mirick, Scott Davis, and David B. Thomas, "Antiperspirant Use and the Risk of Breast Cancer," *Journal of the National Cancer Institute* 94.20 (October 16, 2002): 1578.
3. Marilie D. Gammon, et al., "The Long Island Breast Cancer Study Project: a description of a multi-institutional collaboration to identify environmental risk factors for breast cancer," *Breast Cancer Research and Treatment* 74 (Kluwer Academic Publishers, 2002): 235–254.
4. "Long Island Study Finds No Link Between Pollutants and Breast Cancer," *Journal of the National Cancer Institute* 94.18 (September 18, 2002): 1348–1351.
5. Breast Cancer Progress Review Group, "Charting the Course: Priorities for Breast Cancer Research, Conclusions," *National Cancer Institute* (November 25, 2001), http://prg.nci.nih.gov/breast/bprgconclusions.html, accessed 14 February 2003.

CHAPTER 45
1. Cathy Dunn, "Gifts from the Sea," *CURE*, 1.4 (December 2002): 65.

BIBLIOGRAPHY

Althouse, Valere and Larry. *You Can Save Your Breast*. New York: W.W. Norton & Company, Inc., 1982.

Antman, Karen. "When Are Bone Marrow Transplants Considered?" *Scientific American* 275.3 (September, 1996): 124.

Bazell, Robert. *Her-2*. New York: Random House, 1999.

Bond, Laura, "Dogged Determination," a profile on Harriette Grober, MAMM (May, 2001): 53.

Brinker, Nancy G. *The Race Is Run One Step at a Time: Every Woman's Guide to Taking Charge of Breast Cancer and My Personal Story*. Arlington, Texas: The Summit Publishing Group, 1995.

Gaynes, Fanny. *How Am I Gonna Find a Man If I'm Dead?* Wayne, PA: Morgin Press, 1994.

Gorman, Christine. "Rethinking Breast Cancer," *Time* (February 18, 2002): 50.

Hirshaut, Yashar and Peter I. Pressman. *Breast Cancer: The Complete Guide*. New York: Bantam Books, 2000.

Kushner, Rose. *Breast Cancer: A Personal History and Investigative Report*. New York and London: Harcourt Brace Jovanovich, 1975.

Landau, Elaine. *Breast Cancer*. New York: F. Watts, Grolier Publishing, 1995.

Lee, John R., M.D., David Zava, Ph.D., and Virginia Hopkins. *What Your Doctor May Not Tell You About Breast Cancer: How Hormone Balance Can Help Save Your Life*. New York: Warner Books, 2002.

Leopold, Ellen. *A Darker Ribbon: Breast Cancer, Women and Their Doctors in the Twentieth Century*. Boston: Beacon Press, 1999.

Lerner, Barron H., M.D. *The Breast Cancer Wars*. New York: Oxford University Press, 2001.

Link, John, M.D. *The Breast Cancer Survival Manual*, second edition. New York: Henry Holt and Company, 1998.

Love, Susan, M.D., with Karen Kindsey. *Dr. Susan Love's Breast Book*, third edition. Cambridge: Perseus Publishing, 2000.

Majure, Janet. *Breast Cancer*. Berkeley Heights: Enslow Publishers, 2000.

Middlebrook, Christina. *Seeing the Crab: a memoir of dying*. New York: Basic Books, a division of Harper Collins Publishers, Inc., 1996.

Mitchell, Deborah and Deborah Gordon, M.D. *Breast Health the Natural Way*. New York: John Wiley & Sons, Inc., 2001.

Olivotto, Ivo, M.D., Karne Gelmon, M.D., and Urve Kuusk, M.D. *Breast Cancer: All you need to know to take an active part in your treatment*, second edition. Vancouver: Intelligent Patient Guide, 1998.

Pharmaceutical Research and Manufacturers of America. *New Medicines in Development for Cancer*. Washington, D.C., 2001.

Rollin, Betty. *First You Cry*. New York: Quill, imprint of Harper Collins Publishers, 1976.

Schofield, Lisa. "Soy Isoflavones." *Vitamin Cottage Health Hotline* (October 2001).

Schofield, Jill R., M.D. and William Robinson, M.D., Ph.D. *What You Really Need to Know About Moles and Melanoma*. Baltimore: Johns Hopkins University Press, 2000.

Shaffer, Marianne L., R.N. *Bone Marrow Transplants*. Dallas: Taylor Publishing Co., 1994.

Shamsuddin, AbulKalam M., M.D., Ph.D. *IP-6 Nature's Revolutionary Cancer Fighter*. New York: Kensington Books, 1998.

Sproull, Amy, et al. *A Breast Cancer Journey: Your Personal Guidebook from the Experts at the American Cancer Society*. American Cancer Society, 2001.

Stabiner, Karen. *To Dance with the Devil: The New War on Breast Cancer*. New York: Delacorte Press, 1997.

Wittman, Juliet. *Breast Cancer Journal, a century of petals*. Golden: Fulcrum Publishing, 1993.

ABOUT THE AUTHOR

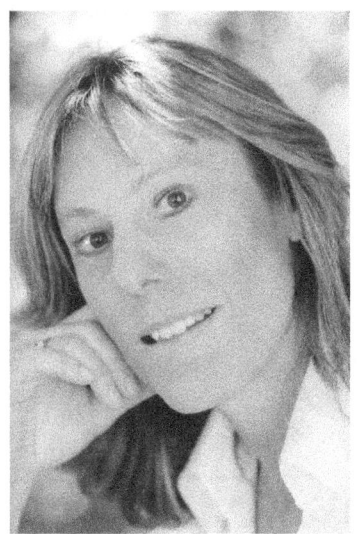

Diane Lane Chambers has a degree in Therapeutic Recreation from the University of Colorado and is a nationally certified sign language interpreter. From her work as an interpreter she wrote her first book, *Words in My Hands: A Teacher, A Deaf-Blind Man, An Unforgettable Journey* (Ellexa Press LLC, 2005).

As a breast cancer advocate, Diane is an active member of the National Breast Cancer Coalition. She is a 2003 graduate of the Coalition's Project LEAD and since then has participated in a number of the NBCC's Advocacy Trainings in Washington, D.C., and Lobby Days on Capitol Hill. In December 2005 she attended the San Antonio Breast Cancer Symposium and graduated from the Alamo Breast Cancer Patient Advocate Program. Locally, she volunteers for the American Cancer Society, giving presentations and meeting with newly diagnosed women as part of the Reach to Recovery Program. She lives with her husband Jim in Conifer, Colorado.

www.ingramcontent.com/pod-product-compliance
Lightning Source LLC
Chambersburg PA
CBHW050619300426
44112CB00012B/1568